COMMUNICATING
WITH
DEAF PEOPLE

Communicating with Deaf People: A Resource Manual for Teachers and Students of American Sign Language by Harry W. Hoemann, Ph.D., is a volume in the PERSPECTIVES IN AUDIOLOGY Series—Lyle L. Lloyd, Ph.D., series editor. Other volumes in this series include:

Published:

Language Development and Intervention with the Hearing Impaired by Richard R. Kretschmer, Jr., Ed.D., and Laura W. Kretschmer, Ed.D.

Noise and Audiology, edited by David M. Lipscomb, Ph.D.

Supervision in Audiology by Judith A. Rassi, M.A.

Auditory Management of Hearing-Impaired Children: Principles and Prerequisites for Intervention edited by Mark Ross, Ph.D., and Thomas G. Giolas, Ph.D.

In Preparation:

Elements of Hearing Science edited by Lawrence J. Deutsch, Ph.D., and Alan M. Richards, Ph.D.

Psychology of Deafness by Harry W. Hoemann, Ph.D.

Rehabilitative Audiology (Part I: The Adult/Part II: The Elderly Client) edited by Raymond H. Hull, Ph.D.

Introduction to Instrumental Phonetics by Colin Painter, Ph.D.

A Primer of Acoustic Phonetics by J. M. Pickett, Ph.D.

Hearing Assessment edited by William F. Rintelmann, Ph.D.

American Sign Language and Sign Systems by Ronnie Bring Wilbur, Ph.D.

Publisher's Note

Perspectives in Audiology is a carefully planned series of clinically oriented, topic-specific textbooks. The series is enriched by contributions from leading specialists in audiology and allied disciplines. Because technical language and terminology in these disciplines are constantly being refined and sometimes vary, this series has been edited as far as possible for consistency of style in conformity with current majority usage as set forth by the American Speech and Hearing Association, the *Publication Manual of the American Psychological Association,* and *The University of Chicago Manual of Style.* University Park Press and the series editors and authors welcome readers' comments about individual volumes in the series or the series concept as a whole in the interest of making Perspectives in Audiology as useful as possible to students, teachers, clinicians, and scientists.

A Volume in the Perspectives in Audiology Series

COMMUNICATING WITH DEAF PEOPLE

A Resource Manual for Teachers and Students of American Sign Language

by
Harry W. Hoemann, Ph.D.

Associate Professor
Department of Psychology
Bowling Green State University

With illustrations by
Shirley A. Hoemann

University Park Press
Baltimore

UNIVERSITY PARK PRESS
International Publishers in Science and Medicine
233 East Redwood Street
Baltimore, Maryland 21202

Copyright © 1978 by University Park Press

Typeset by Shannon Typographic Services
Brodbecks, Pa.

Manufactured in the United States of America by
The Maple Press Company

419

Library of Congress Cataloging in Publication Data

Hoemann, Harry W.
Communicating with deaf people.

(Perspectives in audiology series)
Includes bibliographical references and index.
1. Sign language. I. Title. II. Series.
[DNLM: 1. Deafness — Rehabilitation. 2. Manual
communication. HV2474 H694c]
Hv2474.H64   419   78-17193
ISBN 0-8391-1259-9

to Jan MacMichael Sandgren

CONTENTS

PREFACE TO PERSPECTIVES IN AUDIOLOGY

Audiology is a young, vibrant, dynamic field. Its lineage can be traced to the fields of education, medicine, physics, and psychology in the nineteenth century and the emergence of speech pathology in the first half of this century. The term "audiology," meaning the science of hearing, was coined by Raymond Carhart in 1947. Since then, its definition has expanded to include its professional nature. Audiology is the profession that provides knowledge and service in the areas of human hearing and, more broadly, human communication and its disorders. As evidence of the growth of audiology as a major profession, in the 1940's there were no programs designed to prepare "audiologists," while now there are over 112 graduate training programs accredited by the Education and Training Board of the American Board of Examiners in Speech Pathology and Audiology for providing academic and clinical training designed to prepare clinically competent audiologists. Audiology is also a major area of study in the professional preparation of speech pathologists, speech and hearing scientists, and otologists.

Perspectives in Audiology is the first series of books designed to cover the major areas of study in audiology. The interdisciplinary nature of the field is reflected by the scope of the volumes in this series. The volumes currently in preparation (see p. ii) include both clinically oriented and basic science texts. The series consists of topic-specific textbooks designed to meet the needs of today's advanced level student. Each volume will also serve as a focal reference source for practicing audiologists and specialists in many related fields.

The Perspectives in Audiology series offers several advantages not usually found in other texts, but purposely featured in this series to increase the practical value of the books for practitioners and researchers, as well as for students and teachers.

1. Every volume includes thorough discussion of all relevant clinical and/or research papers on each topic.
2. Every volume is organized in an educational format to serve as the main text or as one of the main texts for graduate and advanced undergraduate students in courses on audiology and/or other studies concerned with human communication and its disorders.
3. Unlike ordinary texts, **Perspectives in Audiology** volumes will retain their professional reference value as focal reference sources for practitioners and researchers in career work long after completion of their studies.
4. Each volume serves as a rich source of authoritative up-to-date information and valuable reviews for specialists in many fields, including administration, audiology, early childhood studies, linguistics, otology, psychology, pediatrics, public health, special education, speech pathology, and speech and hearing science.

Currently the habilitation of hearing-impaired persons is encompassing a broad repertiore of approaches that includes the use of manual communication, particularly American Sign Language (ASL), by deaf people. Therefore, it is vital that persons working with signing members of the deaf community have a better understanding of ASL and are themselves able to communicate fluently in it. *Communicating with Deaf People: A Resource Manual for Teachers and Students of American Sign Language,* by Harry W. Hoemann, is designed with these objectives in mind.

This volume provides the practical, direct application of recent ASL research in the teaching and learning of ASL. A forthcoming volume, *American Sign Language and Sign Systems*, by Ronnie Bring Wilbur, presents the basic linguistics of ASL and other sign systems. The two volumes together form an up-to-date study of ASL theory and application. They also reflect the broad scope of the **Perspectives in Audiology** series, which encompasses both basic research and application.

Communicating with Deaf People: A Resource Manual for Teachers and Students of American Sign Language is an applied book with practical exercises. Through its use, those whose primary means of communication is spoken English will better understand native users of ASL and will become more proficient in the use of ASL. As a result, it is hoped, they will be better able to provide habilitative services to hearing-impaired individuals.

Lyle L. Loyd, Ph.D.
Chairman and Professor of Special Education
Professor of Audiology and Speech Sciences
Purdue University

FOREWORD

Anyone who has invested time in numerous sign language classes only to discover that even the simplest conversation with a native signer is beyond his/her ability will recognize and appreciate the need for *Communicating with Deaf People: A Resource Manual for Teachers and Students of American Sign Language*, by Harry W. Hoemann. As more linguistic information becomes available, the differences between signs in class and signs in real context becomes increasingly apparent. To this end, the presentation of such information to sign language teachers begins to fill a tremendous gap. Instead of requiring memorization of first the fingerspelling alphabet, then isolated lists of signs, then signs in English word order, the utilization of recent linguistic information and second language teaching techniques should overhaul both the content and the procedures in sign language classes. The inclusion of facial expression, modification in space, reduplication for grammatical purposes, and other changes in signs that result from the context in which they are placed may be seen as a divergence from the traditional teaching approach.

As a beginning, it must be recognized that a native signer is not necessarily qualified to be a teacher of sign language any more than any one of us could teach the basic principles of gravity even though each time we let go of an object it falls toward the center of the earth, nor could we teach anatomy even though we all have bodies, nor for that matter would the schools allow any of us to teach public school English without the proper certification, even though most of us are native speakers of English. Perhaps the best example, one with which most of us have had some experience, is the training of students to teach French, Spanish, or German. First they learn the language, then study the structure, then read the literature, then take methods of teaching courses, then undergo supervised student teaching, and finally obtain some form of certification at the state level. In the same sense, American Sign Language is a modern language, and the teachers of ASL should be at least as qualified as teachers of any other modern language, or as Ingram (1977) put it: "Good intentions do not erase bad results." Thus, while we are all interested in seeing that more people learn sign language and use it for the benefit of deaf children and adults alike, we would also like to see the best possible teaching job with the best possible communicative skills resulting. The Sign Instructor's Guidance Network (S.I.G.N.) has recently been formed in the United States to develop and maintain competencies for teachers of sign language. Although the competencies are still being formulated, knowledge of ASL linguistic structure and of various approaches to second language teaching are most assuredly high on the list.

Ingram (1977) reviewed a number of second language teaching approaches that have been used for spoken languages. These include (1) the grammar-translation method, which was taught by recitation, dictionary usage, parts of speech, memorization of declensions, conjugations, and grammar rules, and which was "a dismal flop"; (2) the direct method, which banned the first language from the classroom and put the student in meaningful situations in which the second language could be used and practiced; (3) the audiolingual method, in which the emphasis was removed from learning about the language, to "establish as habits the patterns" of the language, rather than individual sentences, by means of pattern drill; (4) the cognitive-code method, which cycled back to the inclusion of teaching about the language, based on the generative-transformational assumption that language learning and use required knowledge of the underlying phonological, morphological, and syntactic rules of language; and (5) the semiotic method, which considers language to be another form of cultural behavior, and which emphasizes the social activity and context that surround and affect language use. Ingram also outlined "the progressive approach" for sign language teaching, which contains the following phases: "[1] a preparatory phase, in which students are acclimated to communication in the manual-visual mode, [2] instruction in ASL . . . with primary emphasis on the development of comprehension rather than production, [3] instruction in fingerspelling, using a phonetic or 'cluster' method, [4] further instruction in ASL, [5] instruction in simultaneous communication, and [6] instruction in Manual English" (Ingram, 1977: 17-18).

Dennis Cokely, in his foreword to Hoemann (1976), discussed a number of principles that should be considered for teaching ASL. These include: "[1] There should be a period of readiness and preparation for learning the language. [2] Development of receptive skills in ASL should precede receptive skills. [3] Fingerspelling should be taught relatively late in an ASL course. [4] There should be a deaf informant in every ASL course. [5] Students should be exposed to as wide a variety of signers as possible. [6] Care should be exercised in the selection of materials for a course in ASL" (Cokely, 1975: viii-ix).

In addition to such procedural considerations, the teacher of ASL must also be conscious of the structure of ASL. There are, for example, linguistic constraints that govern such things as ASL word order or allowable combinations of sign parts into a single or compound sign (such as combining the handshape from one sign with the movement or place of formation of another sign). When a student produces an ungrammatical sentence, the teacher must be able to correct it, exactly as one would expect a teacher of any other modern language to do. It is necessary to emphasize Cokely's and Hoemann's cautions: check with a native signer.

All of this information, much of which is readily available, would remain scattered but for the initial guiding framework now provided by this book. The need for adequate knowledge about ASL content is easy to demonstrate; one of my sign language teachers told the class that ASL has no verbs. This and other misconceptions, such as ASL has no word order or has "ungrammatical" word order, and the neglect of facial expression, movement in space, various means of pronominalization, verb inflection, and other grammatical processes in ASL are errors that cannot be perpetuated. There is a body of knowledge that the qualifed teacher of sign language should have. Aspects of this knowledge are introduced in each of the chapters in this book and provide the interested reader with a sufficient background to proceed with the more detailed linguistic descriptions given elsewhere. The reference list provides numerous sources of information on ASL structure. Recent books also cover ASL structure in varying ways, for example, Klima and Bellugi (in press), Siple (in press), and Wilbur (1978; in press). Older books should not be ignored: Fant (1972), Madsen (1972), and Hoemann (1976). To keep up to date, *Sign Language Studies* should be considered, as well as the National Symposium on Sign Language Research and Teaching, which seems to be turning into an annual event.

By helping to better prepare teachers of sign languages, Hoemann is contributing to better communication with deaf children and adults through more fluent parents, audiologists, teachers of the hearing impaired, and other professionals who serve the deaf community. Eventually, larger numbers of deaf individuals whose primary language is ASL will benefit from his effort.

REFERENCES

Cokely, D. 1975. Foreword to Hoemann (1975), vii-x.

Fant, L. 1972. *Ameslan: An Introduction to American Sign Language.* National Association of the Deaf, Silver Spring, Md.

Hoemann, H. 1976. *The American Sign Language: Lexical and Grammatical Notes with Translation Exercises.* National Association of the Deaf, Silver Spring, Md.

Ingram, R. 1977. *Principles and Procedures of Teaching Sign Languages.* The British Deaf Association, Carlisle, England.

Klima, E., and U. Bellugi. *The Signs of Language.* Harvard University Press, Cambridge, Mass. In press.

Madsen, W. 1972. *Conversational Sign Language II: An Intermediate Manual.* Gallaudet College Press, Washington, D.C.

Siple, P. *Understanding Language through Sign Language Research.* Academic Press, New York. In press.

Wilbur, R. (ed.). 1978. *Sign Language Research.* A special issue of *Communication and Cognition.*

Wilbur, R. *American Sign Language and Sign Systems: Research and Applications.* University Park Press, Baltimore. In press.

Ronnie Bring Wilbur, Ph.D.
Assistant Professor
School of Education
Department of Special Education
Boston University

PREFACE

This book was written for teachers and students of American Sign Language who wish to acquaint themselves with the growing body of information about structural features of the language. This information is available in numerous conference papers and professional journals, but pulling some of it together into one place seemed to be a useful thing to do. Moreover, since the original sources generally presuppose prior knowledge of some technical jargon, it also seemed desirable to prepare an introduction to this literature that guides the reader gently toward a mastery of both the terminology and the concepts to which it refers.

Right now there seems to be an explosion of knowledge about American Sign Language. Teachers and students who are aware of the research activity that is going on are clearly desirous of access to this information. Both teaching and learning ought to benefit from an understanding of the variety of strategies by which meaning is coded in American Sign Language. I am pleased to have this opportunity to share with my fellow teachers and students of Sign the exciting challenge of exploring some of its various resources as a linguistic system.

Harry W. Hoemann, Ph.D.

ACKNOWLEDGMENTS

A great many people made this publication possible. Acknowledgments must include, first, the deaf linguistic community, whose members have developed and preserved ASL as a linguistic system. Equally important for students of ASL, members of the deaf community have always been willing to share their language with hearing persons whom they have come to know as friends. Second, deserving of mention are the several hundred students at Bowling Green State University who have shared with me the rewarding adventure of studying ASL together. Third, I commend the scholars whose research findings are reflected in this volume. Two of them, Charlotte Baker and Ronnie Wilbur, graciously contributed critical reviews of the manuscript prior to its publication. The contents also benefited from helpful comments made by Joan Forman. Of course, these good people should not be held responsible for the published version.

Finally, I wish to thank the several agencies and organizations at Bowling Green State University that have supported the teaching of Sign language on this campus, including WBGU-TV, The Faculty Development Program Implementation Committee, the Bowling Green State University Foundation, Inc., The Instructional Media Center, the Computational Services Center, and The Department of Psychology.

The book is dedicated to Jan MacMichael Sandgren, a former Bowling Green student who first encouraged me to begin teaching Sign language on the Bowling Green campus.

INTRODUCTION

The information presented in this volume is intended to make teaching and learning Sign more interesting, more fun, and somewhat easier than it has been before. The interest value comes from explicit treatment of features of American Sign Language (ASL) that seem to be all but invisible even to native signers until they are subjected to linguistic analysis. The fun comes from the sense of mastery and accomplishment that can be derived from learning another language, especially one in which one's body and soul can be put into the message. And any time a subject to be learned is made more interesting and more fun, it also seems somehow to have been made easier.

WHAT IS AMERICAN SIGN LANGUAGE?

Making ASL easier to teach and to learn has not meant simplifying the subject matter. Indeed, the scope of what needs to be covered has been greatly enlarged from the content of what once passed for a Sign Language Class (Fant, 1977; Hoemann, 1977; Ingram 1977). Some still-current myths need to be exposed (Markowicz, 1977), and some classroom practices need to be revised. No longer can a teacher of ASL show students how to execute a list of signs from an illustrated book, make some educated guesses as to why the signs are made the way they are, test the students' memory for signs presented in previous classes, and call it a night. Students need to be shown how an infinite variety of meanings can be coded in Sign and how ASL sentences are structured grammatically. Students need to learn how signs are modified in their actual use so as to reflect either linguistic or situational constraints. They need to learn how certain modulations reliably affect the meaning of certain signs and how much freedom a signer has to alter the execution of a sign for a literary or rhetorical effect. None of this information is to be found in the published picture books depicting the vocabulary of ASL. Unless it is explained that the pictured signs are "citation forms," that is, models of an idealized or formalized execution, such texts can be very misleading to the student of ASL.

Sign, or Ameslan (ASL), is the language system used by over half a million deaf persons in the United States and Canada. Its historical roots go back at least in part to French Sign Language and to the Institute for the Deaf and Dumb in Paris, where Thomas Hopkins Gallaudet obtained both some supervised practice in teaching the deaf and the services of a deaf instructor, Clerc, for the school that was to be founded in the United States at Hartford, Connecticut (Frishberg, 1975; Lane, 1976, 1977; Stokoe, 1974; Woodward, 1976b, 1976c). Sign is the language most likely to be acquired spontaneously by deaf children in North America from peer and adult models. Its current status is assured by the strength of the deaf linguistic community, for whom the use of ASL serves as a defining characteristic (Croneberg, 1965a; Furth, 1973; Markowicz, 1972; Markowicz and Woodward, in press; Meadow, 1972; Moores, 1972). Indeed, one can sense among deaf people a rising tide of "deaf pride" and "deaf power" in their growing respect for and knowledge of their language of Sign (Fleischer, 1977; Kannapell, 1974, 1977; Lentz, 1977; Padden, 1977).

Sign has a grammar and a lexicon that can be learned and taught as a second language for hearing persons who speak English.

Needless to say, a teacher of ASL should be fairly fluent in the language. Something very close to native competence is desirable. The Sign Instructor's Guidance Network (O'Rourke, 1977) is developing certification procedures that will help to ensure that teachers of ASL know ASL.

But knowledge of the language is not enough. Over two hundred million people in the United States and Canada know English. This does not qualify them to teach English professionally. By the same token, having had deaf parents may ensure that a person knows ASL, but it does not ensure that the person knows how to teach. Teachers of ASL must be able to lay claim to credentials over and above fluency in the language (Cross, 1977; Ingram, 1977).

ASL *VS* ENGLISH

Since hearing persons in the United States already know English, it is a great temptation for them to: (1) learn signs as if they stood for English words, and (2) structure Sign language sentences in the word order of English sentences. Many adventitiously or well educated deaf people also sign in English, especially to hearing persons, partly because English is a language with higher status than Sign in the United States and partly because hearing persons have a great deal of difficulty understanding ASL. Stokoe (1971, 1972) has described the diglossic continuum which characterizes ASL usage in the United States (see also Woodward, 1973). This continuum is said to range from signed English (the H end of the scale) to colloquial ASL or Ameslan (the L end of the scale). Related to the high social status associated with signed English and, perhaps, even partly responsible for it, is the commitment of the educational establishment to the teaching of English (Bonvillian and Charrow, 1972; Bonvillian, Charrow, and Nelson, 1973; Mindel and Vernon, 1971; Moores, 1972, 1977).

Since educational institutions have a vested interest in teaching English, they have sometimes sponsored Sign language instructional programs whose subject matter was not the ASL usage of deaf persons but rather one of the language intervention systems, such as Seeing Essential English (SEE 1) (Anthony, 1971), Signing Exact English (SEE 2) (Gustason, Pfetzing and Zawoklow, 1972), or Signed English for Preschoolers (Bornstein, Saulnier, and Hamilton, 1976).

This manual was written for teachers who wish to make deaf usage the model of what to teach and what needs to be learned. This means that it presupposes that the teacher is a fluent user of ASL and has access to the deaf linguistic community for knowledge about ASL usage. Second, this manual was written for teachers, intermediate and advanced students, and others with a basic knowledge of Sign who want to know something about ASL on a more formal level. This latter aim requires attention to materials that have not ordinarily been included in a Sign language class.

AVAILABLE INSTRUCTIONAL MATERIALS

Louie Fant (1972) made the first major departure from traditional approaches to teaching ASL when he authored *Ameslan: An Introduction to American Sign Language*. There, for the first time, students of Sign were given whole sentences in ASL instead of isolated signs. The Sign language instructional program at

Bowling Green State University made use of the *Ameslan* text and later supplemented it with an additional text, *American Sign Language: Lexical and Grammatical Notes with Translation Exercises* (Hoemann, 1976).

The present volume is offered for those who prefer a topical treatment of issues that were treated in the context of translations from English to Sign in the former texts. Together with other scholarly treatments of ASL they should provide teachers with a wealth of materials from which to draw for the preparation of lesson plans for a Sign language class. A teacher of ASL should never have to go to class wondering what to do with the available time. Students, too, should no longer need to wonder what it is that they are trying to learn how to do. The available instructional materials and their accompanying films and videotapes are beginning to provide a more and more adequate model of what ASL is and, therefore, what it is that needs to be learned.

It takes a considerable amount of courage for one teacher to advise another how to go about the teaching task. Regardless of what is said or written down, something else could have been said or written down, instead. Morever, there is always the chance that someone can dismiss what has been said as useless or lacking in value. But the same can be said for an art museum, a Broadway production, or a baseball lineup. Just about everything that is done could have been done differently, and one way will please one person and another way will please another.

In the case of ASL, it is extraordinarily hazardous to venture statements that should sound at all authoritative. Many of the details of ASL have yet to be analyzed systematically or reduced to a formal description. Even the topics that have been researched have been studied by, at most, one or two investigators. Independent replications and confirmations of the findings are lacking. Many of the research reports cited in the literature were presented at conferences attended only by other linguists. Unless the proceedings were published, the papers are accessible only through private circulation. Forty percent of the references to Sign language publications in Friedman's recent text (1977b) are not in the public domain. One need not take anything away from the competencies of the pioneers in the field of Sign language study to concede that teachers are currently required to take a great deal on faith. They have only their own personal experiences and observations to reassure them that the "discoveries" of the linguists have been there all along if only one had the ability to see them.

This "Of course!" phenomenon is rather reassuring. I have attended several conferences in which a linguist was expounding on some syntactic feature of ASL to a deaf and hearing audience, and I have yet to see a time when the deaf persons in the audience began shaking their heads in disbelief at the description they were being given of their language. On the contrary, audience response is more likely to take the form of surreptitious practice of the examples being presented followed by comments like TRUE or RIGHT.

But how are teachers of ASL to benefit from the insights generated by linguists and psycholinguists? Scholarly research is often couched in technical jargon that is intimidating even to fellow researchers trained in other disciplines. Unfortunately, most researchers do not take the trouble to translate their own findings into common, ordinary prose. And if they do not, who will?

Whether they wish to or not, teachers must. It is their job. And it is not a trivial assignment. It takes more than a little skill to read published research with a critical eye, to evaluate the quality of the data, to judge the tenability of the conclusions, to assess the implications of the results. An uncritical acceptance of everything that passes for Sign language research today would be just as indefensible for a teacher as to ignore it all as if it had never happened. The teacher of ASL, therefore, faces a worthy challenge, first to understand and to evaluate what the researchers are saying about ASL; second, to judge, from all that is said, what is worth sharing with their students; and finally, to present this information in a form that students can grasp and use on their way to learning the language.

OUTSIDE LEARNING EXPERIENCES

It seems fairly clear that if the only learning of Sign occurs during class time, then not much is going to be learned. Some outside learning experiences have to be arranged. Optimally the students should be placed in contact with a deaf population so that they can observe Sign in use and practice it with deaf people. If this is not a reasonable possibility, films or videotapes should be provided for the students. It simply is not fair for an instructor to make demands on students that they can fulfill only with difficulty since they are not given reasonable access to the information. Certainly the citation forms of a Sign vocabulary can be made available in a language laboratory or library equipped with film projectors or videotape playback equipment. The 500 *Sign Language Flash Cards* (Hoemann and Hoemann, 1973), for example, are available on 3/4 inch color cassettes or on 1/2 inch black and white reel to reel videotape from WBGU-TV, Bowling Green, Ohio. Film cassettes of O'Rourke's (1973) *A Basic Course in Manual Communication* are available from the National Association of the Deaf (814 Thayer Ave., Silver Spring, Md.). Models of the Sign versions of *American Sign Language* (Hoemann, 1976) are also available from WGBU-TV. Its studios have recently prepared a ''Survival Sign Language'' videotape which provides models of several hundred brief, ordinary, everyday expressions in Sign. Given access to such videotapes, it is not unreasonable to expect students in a beginning 10-week course to master a Sign vocabulary of upwards of 500 signs and to be able to understand the meaning of simple ASL sentences made up of familiar vocabulary.

VOCABULARY QUIZZES

To achieve this result, however, the instructor cannot waste time in class demonstrating how to make isolated citation forms of signs. Let the videotape do that. In class a weekly receptive quiz of 50 to 60 signs drawn randomly from the vocabulary pool will monitor students' progress. Not more than 15 minutes a week should be spent on vocabulary quizzes and feedback. Students can be allowed to grade their own papers on alternate weeks to encourage them to work for mastery of the subject matter rather than for a grade.

TRAINING PERCEPTUAL SKILLS

Early in a course in ASL it may be a good idea to give special attention to training the students' perceptual skills. The sections on ''Emphasis and Stress'' and ''Natural Expressive Gestures'' in this manual could be used for this purpose. The second exercise accompanying ''Natural Expressive Gestures'' encourages students to pay attention to the facial expressions of the signer and to use them as an important source of information about a signed message. It may also be useful to take a sentence like HAVE MONEY and sign it first as a declarative sentence and then again as a question. For the question one may arch the eyebrows, hunch the shoulders, lean forward, and hold the final pose. Students may then be asked to name all the ways in which the second execution differed from the first. The same contrastive strategy can be used to highlight the salient features of numerous other types of grammatical constructions in Sign, e.g., conditional sentences, emotionally charged statements, commands, etc.

THE PLACE OF FINGERSPELLING

Many classes in ASL begin with one or more lessons on the manual alphabet. This is probably not very productive. If it is Sign that the teacher wants the students to learn, allowing them to learn fingerspelling is tantamount to allowing them to circumvent the rationale of the class and to acquire proficiency in a substitute manual mode. This opinion seems to be shared by other teachers of Sign Language (Cokely in Hoemann, 1976; Fant, 1972; Ingram, 1977).

STRESS RECEPTIVE SKILLS

The goal of the Sign language instructional program for which these materials were prepared is to bridge the gap between the deaf linguistic community and hearing persons who want to relate to certain of its members either personally or professionally. Consequently, receptive skills are considered to be relatively more important than expressive skills. Expressive skills should receive some attention. But in a manual mode, it is the hearing person who has the greater handicap. Deaf people are ordinarily far more likely to understand the clumsy Sign language of a hearing person than is a hearing person likely to understand the free-flowing Sign language of a deaf person. In any case, it is generally more important for hearing persons to be able to understand what deaf people have to say than vice versa. The rationale behind all Sign instruction should include an antipaternalistic bias. Let Sign students first learn to understand deaf people. Then it may be permissible for them also to have something to say and to be understood.

TIE ASL INSTRUCTION TO ASL USAGE

Teachers of ASL must be somewhat humble. No one has experienced all that is encompassed by the term "American Sign Language." Only a few of its ethnic and regional dialects have been studied or described (Croneberg, 1965b; Woodward, 1974b, 1976a; Woodward and Erting, 1975; Woodward, Erting, and Oliver, 1976). Indeed, socially restricted signs, such as signs for sexual behavior, are not well known outside the core of the deaf linguistic community (Woodward, 1976d, 1977). All things considered, the teacher of ASL is really able to model only a narrow slice of reality in a Sign class. Students should be cautioned to expect a great deal of variability and heterogeneity among the deaf populations with whom they may eventually associate. The variety and diversity that one finds in ASL usage should be treated as a fascinating feature of a living language (Woodward, Erting, and Oliver, 1976). The teacher should avoid useless arguments over the "right" way to make a sign. Even a "slip of the hand" is potentially deserving of some attention, and "Ameslish" (Bragg, 1973) may be as widely used in the United States as "Ameslan."

This means, of course, that the teacher of ASL will be forever a student of ASL. There is no end to what one can learn about the variety of strategies available in ASL for coding meanings.

BACK TRANSLATION EXERCISES

One of the research strategies developed by psycholinguists for studying target languages about which little is known is "back translation" (Hoemann and Tweney, 1973; Tweney and Hoemann, 1973). Back translation procedures may begin with an English paragraph which features a selected vocabulary and which includes some interesting translation challenges. With the aid of one or more deaf persons, a Sign version may be developed and either committed to memory or recorded on videotape. Then new translators with no prior knowledge of the original may be recruited to translate the Sign version back into English. If the meaning is preserved, the Sign version can be examined to determine what strategy was used successfully to code the meaning. It may need to be emphasized that there is no one "correct" translation for a complex prose passage. There are many permissible translations that are more or less correct. The final choice is often a matter of taste. Back translations can be continued as often as is desired for a thorough understanding of the manner in which the meaning of an original text might be translated into a target language. The procedures are rich in possibilities not only for examining the properties of target languages but also for discovering the properties of translatable prose and for evaluating the relative abilities of translators.

Some translators may have some difficulty getting away from the influence of the English text in preparing a Sign translation. In that case, the ASL translation may omit some features of Sign that are important, and it may include features that are directly attributable to the influence of the English original. If a researcher suspects that this is happening, the back translation procedures can begin with a Sign version as the original, and the first translation effort can go from Sign to English. As an alternative, a picture, such as a Norman Rockwell print, can be used to specify the semantic content of a message. In any case, a careful scholar will always look for independent confirmation of conclusions.

REFERENTIAL COMMUNICATION TASKS

A second research procedure especially useful with children is a referential communication task (Hoemann, 1972; Jordan, 1973). A set of pictures is shown to a subject who will act as sender. One of the pictures is designated as the referent, and the sender is required to describe it so that the receiver can pick it out from the array. The adequacy of the sender's message can be ascertained from the receiver's performance. The task can be made as easy or as difficult as the examiner wishes by varying the number of items in the array and the manner in which they differ from one another. It is a rewarding experience to discover how many successful strategies 12-year-old deaf children might have for describing "three red circles," "the third shortest line," or "the picture with the picnic table in front of the tree and the trash can off to the right." Studies of the acquisition of language and communication skills in young deaf children are as rewarding as they are challenging (Hoffmeister, Moores, and Ellenberger, 1973; Schlesinger and Meadow, 1972).

HAVE FUN

It can be a lot of fun exploring facets of ASL among deaf populations and sharing new discoveries with a class. Teaching should be fun. When teachers enjoy teaching, students are more likely to enjoy learning. The preparation for teaching should also be a pleasant experience, since it puts the teacher in close contact with the subject matter that is to be taught. Imagine! One can actually become a better teacher of ASL by spending pleasant moments in the company of one's deaf friends and acquaintances.

NOTHING SUCCEEDS LIKE SUCCESS

Of course, learning is more fun when it is successful. A good teacher will build in many opportunities for Sign language students to succeed. The exercises in this resource manual were prepared with success in mind. All but a very few of them can be carried out with ease. Besides these exercises, there are other things that one can do in class that will ensure a feeling of success in the students.

I use *American Sign Language* (Hoemann, 1976) as a major source of models of ASL prose and vocabulary. But as soon as we have completed Lesson One, at the beginning of the second class session I bring in a brief Sign language conversation, demonstrate it to the class, and then have the students pair off and sign it to each other. The conversation is based on vocabulary found in Lesson One. As soon as the students have completed the conversation, I give a 10-item vocabulary quiz drawn from the conversation. Rarely do students miss any items at all. At most they miss one out of 10. It gives beginning students a great sense of accomplishment to know that they are already able to "say" things in ASL, understand things "said" in ASL, and pass a vocabulary quiz with flying colors after only one class session.

Another classroom exercise that is fairly sure to elicit some successful performances is to cover one of the ASL versions from *American Sign Language* in class, instruct the students to study it on the videotape, and then in a subsequent class meeting, sign selected sentences from the Sign version, asking members of the class to say what they mean. The confidence gained from recognizing familiar sentences will lay a good foundation for dealing with novel sentences constructed from a familiar vocabulary.

HAVE A HAPPY DAY

The rationale proposed here for teaching and learning Sign is one that should generate considerable pleasure and satisfaction from students and teachers alike. It stresses understanding more than rote learning, success more than failure, mastery more than grading, and fun more than obligation. I enjoy teaching Sign this way because it seems to yield good results, even with large classes.

COMMUNICATING
WITH
DEAF PEOPLE

SIGNS AS MEANINGFUL UNITS IN ASL

For a long time the majority view held that Sign* was not a language in the same sense as German, French, and English. Linguistic analysis was considered to be impossible or at least inappropriate for a language that was judged to be "iconic," heavily dependent on pantomime, and lacking the kinds of grammatical structures that are commonly found in English and other well known spoken languages.

Linguistic research conducted within the last few years has turned this opinion around (Bellugi, 1976, 1977; Bellugi and Fischer, 1972; Bellugi and Klima, 1975, 1976; Fischer, 1973, 1974, 1975, 1976; Friedman, 1975, 1976, 1977a, 1977b; Klima, 1975; Klima and Bellugi, 1972, 1974, 1975a, in press; Siple, 1978; Stokoe, 1972, 1975; Wilbur, 1976, in press). It is no longer defensible to exclude ASL from the family of human languages on such grounds. Regularities have been found in ASL at all levels of its formulation, from the development of lexical items (vocabulary) to the construction of well formed ASL sentences (grammar). The laws which govern these regularities are found throughout ASL usage (Wilbur, in press), and they are revealed in a special way when they are violated for the purpose of expressing humor or of inventing a "figure of speech" (Klima and Bellugi, 1975b).

Structure is found in spoken languages at increasingly broader and higher levels of organization. Morphemes are the most basic meaningful units. Words are comprised of one or more morphemes, and as the lexicon of a language they have associated with them identifiable fields of meaning. Sentences mean something else than the sum total of the meanings of their words, and, by virtue of their unique organization of propositions, paragraphs also convey a message that is greater than the sum of their parts.

---

*In keeping with popular usage, the terms "Sign" and "ASL" are used interchangeably to refer to American Sign Language, the means of communication preferred by most deaf people in the United States.

1

Linguistics recognizes the need to approach the study of languages on both microcosmic and macrocosmic levels. One approach has been to see languages as organized on three separate levels, phonology, syntax, and semantics. But the same methodology that gave linguistics a powerful tool for the analysis of spoken languages left it at a loss as far as the study of sign languages was concerned. Since sign languages were not made up of sounds, it was assumed without question that they had no phonology. Where was one to begin?

A milestone in the linguistic analysis of ASL structure was achieved in 1960 when William C. Stokoe, Jr., published a monograph proposing that signs were comprised of a finite number of relatively meaningless aspects which could be combined in a very large number of ways so as to generate a lexicon. This analysis of Sign ascribed to it a property analogous to a phonologic system. Since the aspects of ASL enumerated by Stokoe were formed by human hands instead of by means of voiced sounds, he called them "cheremes" from the Greek *cheir* ("hand"). He called the study of the structure of ASL at this level of organization "cherology." (Some current researchers (Battison, 1973, 1974; Friedman, 1977a, Woodward and Erting, 1976) use the term "phonology" for this aspect of ASL structure without any apologies for its etymology.)

The first chapter of this text is devoted to features of specific signs from ASL. Out of deference to the breakthrough that Stokoe's efforts have provided for the field of linguistics, and out of a need to begin as close as one can to the beginning in discussing important features of ASL, this first section begins with a discussion of the aspects of signs first outlined by Stokoe. Some of the more recent formulations of his model of ASL are discussed, and approaches in this level of ASL organization that seem to be comparable to distinctive features in speech are briefly reviewed.

Chapter Two deals with a property of sign languages that has always seemed to fascinate both students and scholars; iconicity, or the extent to which individual signs resemble what they mean (Bellugi and Klima, 1976; Frishberg, 1975; Hoemann, 1975; Mandell, 1977a). Many signs appear to be influenced in their form or structure by their referent. When the form of the referent motivates the form of the symbol, the symbol is said to be a "motivated" symbol. This is in contrast to all but a very few of the words in spoken languages, which do not resemble their meanings in any structural manner. Onomatopoëia is a noteworthy exception. It should be recognized that calling a sign language "iconic" or "motivated" begs the question, since there are not many empirical data to inform us how deaf persons perceive this aspect of ASL, and such data as do exist suggest that persons unfamiliar with ASL cannot guess the meanings of most of the signs from its lexicon. The heuristic value of using the motivation of signs as a mnemonic device for learning their meanings is discussed.

The third chapter in this section takes on the initialization of signs as a linguistic phenomenon that is deserving of careful study. Borrowings by one language from another are a frequent occurrence, but ASL has a unique kind of borrowing that refers (for those who know English) to an English word by means of an initial letter from the manual alphabet and at the same time retains the location and movement associated with a basic sign from ASL (Battison, 1974, 1977).

Chapter Four takes up another interesting feature of ASL, the fact that certain locations and certain hand configurations connote certain specific meanings. Gender markers are singled out for special treatment. There are signs for the male and female gender (Hoemann and Hoemann, 1973), but certain regions of the face can be marked off to also indicate the male gender or the female gender. In like manner, "mental" signs are executed near the forehead, a bent V connotes difficulty, and the open 8 configuration is associated with verbs denoting affect. Apparently, the structural aspects of signs identified by Stokoe (1960) are not always devoid of meaning; the place where certain signs are executed can itself indicate whether the sign refers to a male or a female person.

Chapter Five introduces the concept of a modulation. The signs that are depicted in the typical sign language "dictionary" are "citation forms," formal models of each sign's basic aspects. These may be modified for rhetorical effect, and they may be altered to reflect their grammatical function or to fit the social circumstances. Some of these modifications and alterations are rule governed, and they must be mastered as a part of the ASL grammatical system. As an illustration of how modulations may work in ASL, Chapter Five takes up pluralization. This is an aspect of ASL that has not been discussed much in print, although a number of scholars are working on the topic more or less independent of one another. It is hazardous to make premature comments on an issue that is still that much up in the air, but now that the reader has been forewarned that this text is only a preliminary statement, perhaps it can be tolerated as a potential stimulus to further research. The fact is that we do not understand exactly how pluralization is accomplished in ASL. It may be that it is accomplished only imperfectly and that a lot of ambiguity is left for the receiver to unravel. It happens in other languages, including English, that a receiver must sometimes infer whether a noun is singular or plural from a knowledge of the sender or of the situation. Perhaps this is also the case in ASL. But students of ASL will want to know how to say something in the plural as well as in the singular, and they need to pick up ASL indicators that a noun has been pluralized. Perhaps this section will help.

Chapter Six discusses compounds. Compounding is found in ASL, and its presence has been used by investigators to document that ASL is a rule-governed language. Many compounds are included in published sign language "dictionaries." It may be useful to the student of ASL to be able to identify a compound when he or she sees one.

Chapter Seven is devoted to fingerspelling. Something must be said about it, and this is as good a place as any. Some instructional materials treat fingerspelling early in a course on ASL (e.g., Babbini, 1974). The main reason this was not done here is that we prefer to play down the importance of fingerspelling as a manual communicative channel between the hearing and the deaf. Nevertheless, fingerspelling is important in its own right as a feature of ASL, since there are initialized signs in ASL that use manual alphabet characters, and there are also finger-spelled loan words in ASL that have been taken on from English (Battison, 1976, 1977).

Chapter Eight presents some examples of incorporation (Bellugi and Fischer, 1972). This is a grammatical feature of ASL that is characterized by a great economy of effort (Mayberry, 1978), since it provides an opportunity to bootleg a great deal of information simply by modifying the execution of existing signs instead of inventing new ones or resorting to paraphrasing.

Chapter Nine drops back to a more practical concern, namely, how to add stress or emphasis to a sign or a statement. The discussion includes additional examples of incorporation.

Chapters Ten and Eleven also deal with topics that have attracted a lot of public interest, namely, natural gestures and pantomime. The treatment given these topics here proceeds from the assumption that, when natural gestures and pantomime are assimilated by a manual system of communicating, they will be likely to exhibit features that partake of the grammar of the manual language. Formal linguistic arguments for this assumption can be found in Kegl and Wilbur (1976).

In this section, other issues could have been included stemming from psychologic considerations such as memory, perception, and child development. Some reference is made in later chapters to relevant research from these problem areas when it is considered useful for the teacher or student of ASL. For an extensive discussion of the interface between ASL and cognitive factors, see Friedman (1977b) and Wilbur in press.

CHAPTER 1

FROM CHEREMES TO DISTINCTIVE FEATURES

In his 1960 monograph, Stokoe proposed that each sign in ASL was composed of three simultaneous aspects, a tabula (TAB), a designator (DEZ), and a signation (SIG), corresponding respectively to the location, hand configuration, and movement associated with the sign. Of course, some signs might involve more than one hand configuration, or they may involve a change from one hand configuration to another. Or a sign may involve a movement from one TAB to another. But there are limits to the number of locations, hand configurations, and movements that can be incorporated in a single sign, and there are rules that govern which of the hands may assume which hand configurations so as to produce a lexical item that is recognizable as part of the ASL system. For example, symmetric signs executed by means of alternating movements (with the rare exception of neologisms like "Total Communication" and "El Paso") have the same hand configuration on both hands (Battison, Markowicz, and Woodward, 1975). Examples of such bilateral conformity are MAYBE, WAR, PEOPLE, STAR, CONVERSATION, VISIT, and JUDGE.* The same rule also applies to symmetric signs executed toward or away from the midline. Examples are DARK, CLOSE, FOOTBALL, DON'T, BUT, and DIVIDE. But when one hand assumes a dominant role, and the other hand becomes, in Stokoe's notation, a TAB, the nondominant hand may assume only a limited number of DEZ, or hand configurations (Battison, 1974; Friedman, 1975). These include the A (PROMISE), C (IN), 5 (AMONG), O (VOTE), G (FROM, TO), and B (AGAINST) handshapes, but not the R, F, V, etc., handshapes. According to Battison, Markowicz, and Woodward (1975), these nondominant handshapes have been found in all sign languages thus far studied, and they are the earliest handshapes acquired by deaf children.

The most important feature of Stokoe's hypothesis about the formational parameters of the ASL lexicon is that the number of aspects that are found is not infinite. He identified 12 TABs, 19 DEZ, and 24 SIGs that he considered to be the set of elements from which all ASL

---

*Throughout the book, a SIGN is orthographically represented by capital letters; its "meaning" is in quotation marks; and the *word* that best translates it is italicized (after Wilbur, 1976, p. 434).

signs were formed. Aspects which look similar (e.g., K and P hand-shapes), but which did not act as "distinctive features" in a contrastive analysis of signs, were judged to be "allochers" of the same chereme.

This system of analysis was used to develop the first American Sign Language dictionary to be constructed on the basis of linguistic princi-ples (Stokoe, Casterline, and Croneberg, 1965). Unlike most of the so-called sign language dictionaries (which are really only picture lexicons), the 1965 dictionary authored by Stokoe and his colleagues at Gallaudet College lists signs in a sequence that is derived from his analysis and by which one can "look up" a sign in the same way that one would use an alphabetic sequence to look up a word in a dictionary of a written language.

Recent publications (Battison, 1973; Battison, Markowicz, and Woodward, 1975; Friedman, 1975, 1977a; Stokoe, 1971, 1972) have offered some modifications of this system without causing any serious problem for its basic rationale. For example, a change in the orientation of the hands is sufficient to distinguish NAME from CHAIR. Also, the system was never intended to deal directly with the organization of ASL on the level of phrases and clauses. Although nonmanual aspects of ASL were anticipated in the treatment given ASL in the 1960 monograph, many questions were left for future study to explore in more detail. But these limitations in scope do not detract from the usefulness of Stokoe's cheremic analysis as a linguistic tool, and Stokoe's contribution to the linguistic study of ASL has clearly been a substantial one. Moreover, it came at a time when there was little or no encouragement from the sci-entific community to embark on such a venture and when many scholars were apparently convinced that it was a fruitless enterprise. Its major weaknesses are that it seems to have underestimated the importance of the contribution made by nonmanual aspects of Sign, such as facial ex-pression (Baker and Padden, 1976, in press), and spatial organization (Liddell, 1976, 1977a, 1977b), and it does not resolve the question as to the extent to which ASL uses iconic imitations to represent continuous, real-world phenomena (DeMatteo, 1976, 1977; Mandell, 1977a).

Stokoe's model has also yielded a notation system that has some utility for communicating information in writing about ASL or for keeping a record on paper of ASL productions (see Siple, 1978, for examples). Stokoe assigned a symbol for each TAB, DEZ, and SIG in his system, and these can be used to denote specific lexical items in ASL. For example, an arc open at the bottom represents the forehead. The symbol, G, represents an extended index finger. The notation, x super-script, represents contact. These three symbols, then, can be combined to form the Sign, THINK. Additional examples are presented in Figure 1.

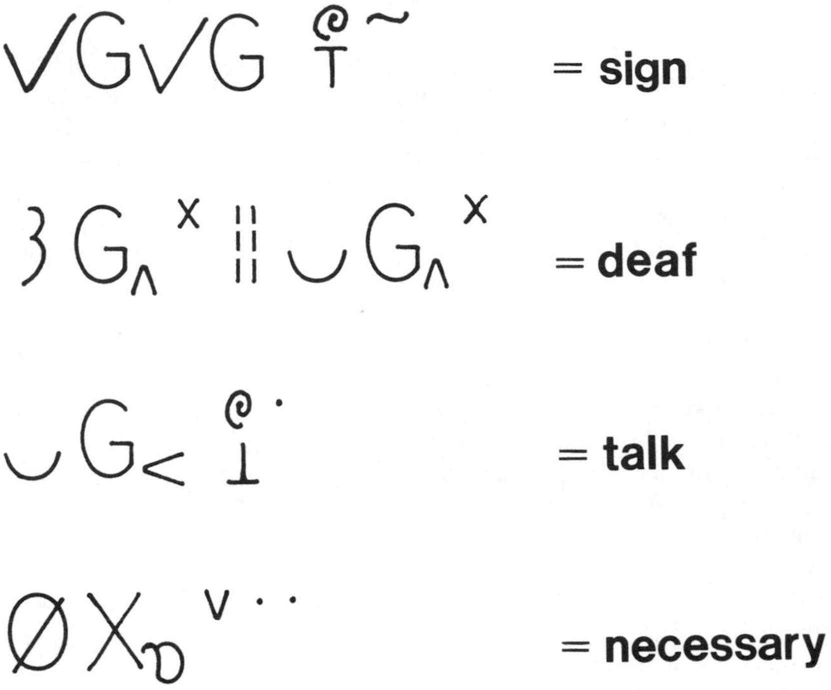

$$\sqrt{G}\sqrt{G} \; \overset{\varrho}{\underset{T}{}} \sim \qquad\qquad = \textbf{sign}$$

$$3\; G_\wedge{}^{X} \; \| \; \cup G_\wedge{}^{X} \qquad = \textbf{deaf}$$

$$\cup G_< \; \overset{\varrho}{\underset{\bot}{}} \; \cdot \qquad\qquad = \textbf{talk}$$

$$\emptyset \, X_{\mathcal{D}} \; {}^{V}{}^{\cdot\cdot} \qquad\qquad = \textbf{necessary}$$

Figure 1. Examples of Stokoe's notation for signs.

Other notation systems have been devised, notably by Peled (n.d.) for Israeli Sign Language and Sutton (1977) for a variety of body movements, including dance, gymnastics, and American Sign Language.

Recent applications of cluster analysis and multidimensional scaling (Hawes, 1976; Lane, Boyes-Braem, and Bellugi, 1976) to features of ASL handshapes have raised the possibility that there are distinctive features in ASL comparable to those that appear to function in spoken languages as a basic set of dimensions enabling users to discriminate one sound from another and one lexical item from another. The absence of nonlinguistic handshapes in the stimulus sets used by these investigators imposes some limits on the conclusions that one may draw from the results. The data may tell us more about the perceptual discriminability of handshapes than about the way in which these handshapes function as part of a linguistic system. Inasmuch as the inexperienced subjects in Hawes' (1976) study generated results similar to the experienced subjects, it appears that knowledge of the language is not necessary for the hypothetical distinctive features to be discriminated.

Stokoe's model of ASL has also provided a basis for a computer simulation (Hoemann, Florian, and Hoemann, 1976). Structural elements identified by Stokoe as basic aspects were stored in a Nova 1220 minicomputer as separate pieces of information, and they were combined by means of subroutines so as to be executed on a graphic display unit. Among the signs that the Nova could execute were MOTHER, FATHER, SUMMER, DRY, and FARM. The information stored in the computer included 11 DEZ , 8 TABs, and 7 SIGs, enough for potentially 616 signs. Over 600 of them were nonsense. It appears that there is a lot of room left in ASL for lexical expansion, and it also appears that most signs differ from one another in more than a single aspect.

Intrusion errors in short-term memory tasks have revealed that signs are coded in memory by deaf persons in terms of the structural aspects originally identified by Stokoe (Bellugi and Klima, 1975; Bellugi, Klima, and Siple, 1975; Siple, Fischer, and Bellugi, 1977). The errors take the form of substituting a permissible TAB, DEZ, or SIG for the correct one. Similar substitutions have been observed to occur in "slips of the hand" in ASL (Bellugi and Klima, 1975). Taken together, these data indicate that signs in ASL are not uniquely different icons, but that they share features which are psychologically meaningful and which may function as distinctive features in the language.

It is reasonable to ask what difference all of this makes for the teaching and learning of Sign. One could argue, for example, that one can learn French without knowing how many phonemes are found in the language or which ones are never found in adjacent positions. But phonology must be reckoned with at some level, and one should be able to spot violations of the phonologic rules of a language. Some of the "new signs" coined by inventors of signed English systems have violated some of the phonologic rules governing the construction of signs. This is not a crime. In fact, the recently coined TOTAL COMMUNICATION violates the rule that symmetric signs should present the same handshape on both hands. But there is strong support within the deaf community for the philosophy referenced by TOTAL COMMUNICATION. Signs that lack such support and that violate phonologic rules are less likely to be accepted by the deaf community in the first place, and if they are accepted, they are likely to be unstable, that is, they are likely to change over time so as to conform to the system.

This latter hypothesis is testable. If a set of "new signs" were invented, half of which conformed to ASL phonologic rules and the other half did not, and if both sets were learned equally well on the basis of an acceptable criterion by fluent users of ASL, it would be predicted that the subjects would show more errors in recall for the nonconforming signs, and that their errors would take the form of modifications in the direction of conformity.

Students of ASL may not need to be able to list all the TABs, DEZ, and SIGs in the system. Indeed, the experts do not agree completely as to the number of each type of "articulatory feature" that may be specified in Sign (Friedman, 1977a; Stokoe, 1960, 1972; Wilbur, in press). But a "feel for the language" (what the Germans call *Sprachgefühl*) requires some awareness of the kinds of sublexical components found in ASL and the amount of freedom one has to modify them when using the language (Frishberg, 1977).

Finally, there may be some value for students, as they commit signs to memory, to take note of those signs which differ in only one aspect (Stokoe's term, 1972) or in only one "articulatory parameter" (Friedman's term, 1977a). Such a contrastive analysis was originally used by Stokoe (1960) to decide which aspects were to be considered cheremes and which were allochers. Knowing which differences in sign executions may result in differences in meaning would seem to be an important thing to know about a language.

EXERCISES

Purpose

To illustrate the utility of Stokoe's cheremic analysis of the structure of signs.

Instructions

Let students generate lists of signs according to the following constraints.

1. List as many signs as you can that use as their TAB the following locations:

   The forehead

   The chin

   The left elbow

2. List as many signs as you can that use as their DEZ the following hand configurations:

   The C hand

The S or A hand (allochers)

The V hand or both V hands

3. List as many signs as you can that use as their movement the following:

A circular motion

A movement forward from the body

A movement downward in front of the body

CHAPTER 2

ICONICITY AND TRANSPARENCY

Teachers of ASL often call attention to the extent to which signs resemble what they mean, since resemblances may help students remember the signs and their meanings (Mandell, 1977a, 1977b). Any strategy that makes it easier for students to learn their lessons is well worth having; consequently, the relationship between the form or appearance of signs and their referents is an appropriate topic to discuss early in a course.

A "motivated" sign is one which in some way resembles what it means. The motivation for some signs (HOUSE, TALK, HEAVY), is so obvious that it can probably be accepted with reasonable certainty as the basis for the origin of the signs. But there is a clear possibility that some explanations for the origins of signs have come about through post hoc speculation. Thus, there are conflicting traditions surrounding the origins of some signs. Is AMERICA a union of states or a split rail fence? PITTSBURGH seems to come from a man reaching into his lapel pocket; but is he reaching for a handkerchief or a cigar? Teachers who use the possible motivations of signs to help students remember them should add the caution that these supposed origins should be taken with a grain of salt.

At one time it was believed that ASL iconicity made it inferior as a language, but this is no longer taken for granted. Scholars are now demanding evidence that iconicity imposes limitations on ASL adequacy before they accept the assumption as a valid one. In any case, the iconicity that fascinates hearing students and learned scholars may be far from obvious to deaf children as they acquire ASL naturally and spontaneously from models in their environment. The very young deaf child who has never seen a cow is not likely to be greatly influenced by the fact that the sign for MILK somewhat resembles the act of milking a cow.

It seems that there is a historical trend toward more abstractness and less iconicity in ASL (Frishberg, 1975, 1976). The motivated aspect drops out as signs lose their idiosyncracies and pantomimic origins. With the passage of time, signs conform more and more to the manner in which other signs are formed. For example, SWEETHEART (see Fig-

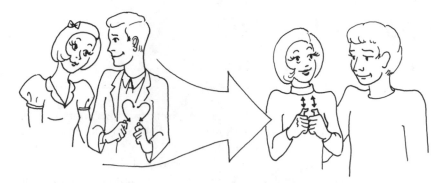

Figure 2. The sign SWEETHEART has changed over time and no longer includes the tracing of a heart on the chest.

ure 2) was once signed by tracing a heart on the chest with the extended thumb of both clenched fists. The sign is now executed in a neutral position, and the movement no longer traces the outline of a heart. Whether this trend is unidirectional and will, one day, lead to the eventual disappearance of almost all iconicity is not clear (Roger Brown, 1977).

As exercise 1 (below) demonstrates, even though some signs are relatively iconic, it does not necessarily follow that their meaning will be transparent to persons who have no prior knowledge of the language. A study of ASL transparency conducted at Bowling Green State University (Hoemann, 1975) revealed that about one-third of the vocabulary was somewhat transparent in meaning to naive observers, one-third was completely opaque, yielding a wide variety of guesses, and one-third was downright misleading, eliciting guesses for which there was a fair amount of consensus but with meanings that were incorrect. Once subjects are told what a sign means, they are often able to pick out an aspect of the referent that seems to have motivated the sign (Bellugi and Klima, 1976). Exercise 2 gives students a feel for this aspect of ASL.

It is all but impossible to predict in advance which aspect of a referent will serve to motivate a sign. Some signs resemble a whole object (AIRPLANE), and some signs resemble a part of an object (DEER). Some signs reflect what a referent does (SCISSORS), and others reflect what one does with the referent (LAWNMOWER). Still others share a little of both kinds of motivation (See Figure 3). COFFEE may be derived from turning a coffee grinder, MILK from milking a cow, and TEA from stirring something in a cup.

Since improvisation is often necessary to translate from English to Sign or to express particular meanings in Sign, students should be given practice in inventing iconic signs (Exercise 3, below). The teacher of

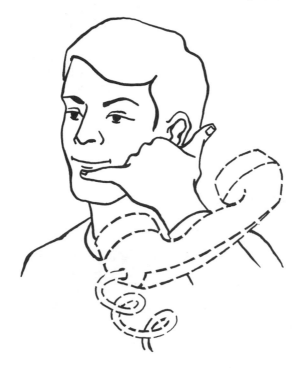

Figure 3. The sign TELEPHONE appears to be motivated both by what it looks like and by what one does with it.

ASL should display an attitude of creative excitement regarding this feature of ASL. Students may benefit from a group discussion of the extent to which their iconic inventions conform to the formational constraints discussed in the previous chapter.

In an extensive essay on iconicity in ASL, Mandell (1977a) has distinguished between *presentation*, in which a referent is indexed (NOSE, BODY, HEAD) or mimed (WRITE, DRINK) and *depiction*, in which a referent is sketched (HOUSE), stamped (MEASLES), or represented by the articulators (TREE, AIRPLANE). Mandell believes that "picture making" is an important aspect of communicating in ASL, and he has provided a tentative description and classification of iconic devices in ASL.

Mandell's essay (1977a) also calls attention to the fact that conventional signs in the ASL lexicon may be either iconic or noniconic; but ad hoc inventions, in order to succeed as a communication, must be sufficiently iconic to allow their meaning to be inferred.

Iconicity provides a dimension of Sign that can be exploited as a literary device. For example, the ears of a donkey can be elongated before bending forward to imply "really stubborn." Iconicity can also add clarity and vividness to a description. For example, an old Victorian house can be given a number of gables of different sizes and levels along with a tower and an ornate front door. Given these literary and rhetorical devices (see Chapter 21), it is clearly an unwarranted assumption that iconicity is a mark of inferiority in a language.

EXERCISES

(1) Purpose

To illustrate the fact that many signs from ASL are not transparent.

Instructions

Students are to guess the meaning of the following signs:

THINK, FINE, MAYBE, RAIN, BORED, FARMER
LETTER, NEW, VISIT, HOME, TIRED, SAY, HOUSE, CAN'T,
    SEE, MOTHER

(2) Purpose

To encourage students to use the motivation of signs as a memory aid.

Instructions

Students are to indicate what aspect of the referent furnishes the motivation for the signs below. Immediately after the exercise, a vocabulary test (Sign to English) can be given to verify that the students now recognize these motivated signs.

FROM, RAIN, TEMPERATURE, GROW, MORNING, THINK, SKY,
    WARM, DRY, DISAPPEAR, PLEASANT
KNOW, BEAUTIFUL, BUILDING, LIKE, FLOWER, TREE, HELP,
    MAYBE, COMPLAIN, HOME

(3) Purpose

To encourage students to innovate and to invent iconic signs to communicate in a manual system.

Instructions

Students are to invent signs for the following (more than one solution is permissible):

1. A man riding a motorcycle
2. A child riding a tricycle
3. A frilly dress
4. A skimpy bathing suit
5. A mirror
6. A newspaper
7. A rail fence
8. A picket fence
9. An ornamental iron fence
10. A mustache (several varieties)

The teacher and students can enlarge upon the list. As an outside assignment, students can prepare a list of referents that can be signed iconically and bring it to class. In the class discussion, the instructor can compare the invented signs with actual signs that are know to exist in ASL.

CHAPTER 3

INITIALIZED SIGNS

A feature of ASL that dates at least as far back as the Abbé de l'Épeé (1776) and his "methodical sign language" is the use of initialization to reference a word from an available spoken language. It is possible that the sign SEARCH, for example, (the right C hand circled in front of the face) references the French, *chercher*. A large number of signs in the published texts on Sign vocabulary (Davis, 1966; Fant, 1964; Hoemann and Hoemann, 1973; Long, 1918; O'Rourke, 1972; Riekehof, 1963; Watson, 1964) are initialized signs. All but a very few of them form the first letter of the English word on the right hand as the sign is executed. An example, PINK from RED, is presented in Figure 4. The result is an

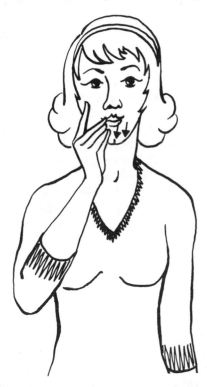

Figure 4. The sign RED may be signed with "P" DEZ for PINK.

extremely complex symbol, which refers to a field of meaning associated with the conventional sign by means of its location and movement, but which, at the same time, refers to an English word and its associated field of meaning by means of its hand configuration. For a discussion of the linguistic status of initialized signs in ASL, see Wilbur (in press).

Such a usage presupposes some bilingual competence on the part of the users of the manual language system. In the absence of knowledge of the English words that the initial letters reference, the field of meaning associated with the sign would have to be developed naturally over a long period of use. In the case of some signs, such as KING, GREEN, WATER, and other common signs, this may indeed have happened for many deaf people. It may be the case that large numbers of deaf children use these initialized signs, know what they mean, but have no idea that the hand configuration has something to do with an English word. One cannot assume that heavy reliance on initialization will induce knowledge of English vocabulary in young deaf children.

Nevertheless, initialized signs are being invented at an unprecedented rate by individuals who believe that such vocabulary expansion will somehow improve upon Sign language as a language and make it a more useful communicative channel for some educational purposes. A noteworthy exception (Paget and Gorman, 1968) is Paget's "New Sign Language," which relied heavily on motivated rather than initialized signs. But the Seeing Essential English (SEE 1)/(Anthony,1971) and the Signing Exact English(SEE2)(Gustason, Pfetzirg, and Zawolkow, 1972), the Signed English for Preschoolers project (Bornstein, 1973, 1974; Bornstein, et al. 1975; Bornstein, Saulnier, and Hamilton, 1976), workshops dealing with rehabilitation and vocational training (Hoemann, 1967, 1970), and manuals published by educational and religious institutions (Bearden and Potter, 1973; Kannapel, Hamilton, and Bornstein, 1969) are replete with entries in their specialized dictionaries that reflect a heavy influence from English as a source language for ASL vocabulary expansion.

Guidelines for the development of technical signs which are compatible with ASL phonology have been developed by teams of researchers at the National Technical Institute for the Deaf (Caccamise, Blasdell, and Bradley, 1977; Caccamise et al., 1977).

Initialization ordinarily causes very little difficulty for the hearing person learning ASL since it ties in directly with a prior knowledge of English. The difficulty arises when the hearing person begins to invent initialized signs or to use some that have been seen in print without first determining whether these signs are known and used by the deaf persons on the receiving end of the communication. The student of ASL should be cautioned that the method has its limitations, and that initialization should not be a favorite device for inventing a new sign for a manual vocabulary. It is better, then, to resort to paraphrase or pantomime so as to avoid undue reliance on the imagination of the receiver to catch the implied English word.

It should be mentioned in passing that some initialized signs use a different letter than the initial one. The sign ARE in the SEE systems, for example, uses the R DEZ with the TAB and SIG of the sign TRULY. The final letter is also sometimes used in addition to the initial letter to distinguish between HIM and HIS.

The student of ASL may benefit from some practice serving on the receiving end of initialized signs. The exercise associated with this chapter is offered as a test of the student's ability to recognize the intended English word from an initialized sign. It is not recommended that the items be learned as new vocabulary. If the exercise proves to be more difficult than expected, this may serve as a warning that initialized signs do not always yield an unambiguous symbol for their referents.

EXERCISES

Purpose
To provide the student with practice recognizing an intended English word from an initialized sign.

Instructions
Sign the following items to the students and have them write down the English word they think is being referenced by the sign. If necessary, indicate the meaning of the original sign ("way," "law," "wise," etc).

1. WAY (initial M on both hands— *method*)
2. LAW (signed with right P hand— *principle*)
3. WISE (signed with right P hand— *philosophy*)
4. DOCTOR (signed with right P hand— *psychiatrist*)
5. LIPREAD (signed with right O hand— *oral*)
6. RED (signed with right P hand— *pink*)
7. THINK (signed with right R hand— *reason*)
8. CLEAN (signed with right P hand— *pure*)
9. LET (initial P on both hands— *permit*)
10. WORD (signed with right V hand— *vocabulary*)

CHAPTER 4

GENDER MARKERS

Gender markers are attached to certain signs in ASL to indicate the difference between male and female gender. Thus, in Sign we can distinguish between a male and a female cousin, a difference that is obscured in English. The distinction between male and female is made in ASL on the basis of separate regions on the face, the forehead and region of the right temple for the male gender and the region of the right cheek and chin for the female gender (see Figure 5).

This is not the only instance in ASL where the location of a group of signs contributes to their semantic content (Mandell, 1977a). "Mental" signs are executed on the forehead (THINK, KNOW, WISE, IGNORANT, FORGET, MISUNDERSTAND, etc.). Emotional signs are executed over the heart (FEEL, PITY, SORRY, GRIEF, etc.). Signs denoting acts of seeing, speaking or eating, or hearing are executed near the eyes, mouth, and ear, respectively.

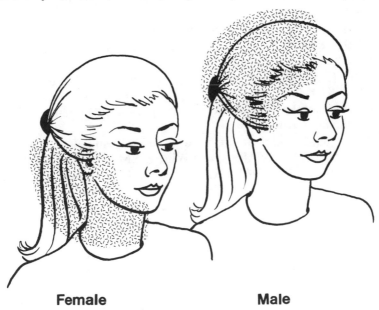

Female   **Male**

Figure 5.   The region of the right cheek and chin serve as the female gender marker, and the region of the forehead serves as the male gender marker.

Handshapes may also connote special meanings. The open 8 hand-shape, which extends the middle finger of the hand, is used for signs involving feeling (FEEL, PITY, SICK, BARE, THRILLED, DE-PRESSED, etc.). The "horns" hand configuration (extended index and little finger) is used for antipathy (MOCK, LAUGH-AT, BETRAY). The bent V is used for difficulty (HARD, STRICT, PROBLEM, DIFFICULT).

These handshapes can be assimilated by other signs with a pre-dictable change in meaning. BORED with "horns" is "terribly bored," and BORED with the open 8 handshape is "bored sick."

Thus, gender markers are only one instance of a more pervasive phenomenon in ASL that allows the location or the hand configuration of a sign to affect a group of signs similarly so as to constitute them as a class.

It is quite possible that the gender markers found in ASL have come down to us from de l'Epeé's (1776) "Methodical Sign Language." Desiring a way to indicate the difference between *le* and *la* in French, de l'Epeé contrived signs for the masculine (indexing the brim of a hat) and the feminine (indexing the bonnet strings down the cheeks), and he applied these gender markers to existing signs from the French Sign Language. This feature of de l'Epee's system for representing in Sign some of the grammatical possibilities of French seems now to have become incorporated in the signs for MOTHER and FATHER, SISTER and BROTHER, NEPHEW and NIECE, SON and DAUGHTER, and several others. Of course, not all signs executed on the forehead are masculine (men will surely disclaim any connotation of gender for the signs DONKEY, STUPID, and FORGET). Nor are all signs executed on the cheek or at the side of the mouth necessarily feminine, such as JEALOUS and SOUR.

These gender markers are used in several compounds, including HUSBAND (MALE + MARRY) and WIFE (FEMALE + MARRY), SON (MALE + BABY) and DAUGHTER (FEMALE + BABY), BROTHER (MALE + SAME), and SISTER (FEMALE + SAME). In these in-stances, not only the region of the face but also the appropriate hand configuration is required.

Far from posing a problem for students of Sign, the efficiency of the gender marker will probably be appreciated, since it reduces the number of signs that need to be learned for a number of kinship signs.

EXERCISES

Purpose

To acquaint students with the use of the gender marker in Sign and assist them in mastering a small vocabulary of kinship signs.

Instructions

Indicate for the students the hand configuration and movement of each of the following signs and let the students execute them in the appropriate location for the gender marker.

1. MAN (adult), WOMAN (adult)
2. BOY (small), GIRL (small)
3. MOTHER, FATHER
4. HUSBAND, WIFE
5. GRANDFATHER, GRANDMOTHER
6. SON, DAUGHTER
7. NEPHEW, NIECE
8. UNCLE, AUNT
9. COUSIN (male), COUSIN (female)
10. BROTHER, SISTER

CHAPTER 5

PLURALIZATION

Languages do not always mark singulars and plurals unambiguously. In English, for example, we do not know whether Bo Peep lost one sheep or more than one until we are told that she did not know where to find *them*. The noun-pronoun agreement in number that is required in English solves the riddle for us.

In ASL it also happens from time to time that the receiver needs some help from the sender in making singulars and plurals unambiguous. The sender ordinarily has a number of options. Consider the following sentence:

The soldiers stood under the tree.

There are at least three ways to mark the noun SOLDIERS as a plural. One is to add the sign for GROUP, generally after the noun that is to be pluralized. The size of the group can be indicated roughly by the size of the sign, GROUP. An exaggerated sign would imply a rather large group. If this is the meaning the signer wants to convey, it is a good choice for a pluralization strategy, since the sign can incorporate information about the size of the group along with the information that it is plural.

Another sign that can be used to pluralize a noun by adding it after the noun is probably best translated *hoard*. It is used infrequently because it is a very strong term, implying a surprisingly large number of items. It is executed by moving both claw hands, palms down, forward from the body. The sign may be executed outward from the face with the eyes squinting as if one can hardly see through the large number of items represented by the forward moving fingers.

Of course, any time an adjective like MANY, FEW, SOME, ALL, FIVE, FIFTEEN, etc., is added to a noun, the noun is construed as a plural. Thus, as in any language, when it is important to make sure that the receiver does not construe a plural as a singular, ASL has a way to make it clear. One obvious way is to modify the noun with a pluralizing adjective. Or, if it is to be emphasized that a noun is singular, ONE can be added as a modifier.

A second pluralization strategy is to use reduplication with the verb along with some spatial organization. Consider again the sentence:

The soldiers stood under the tree.

If the verb, STAND, is executed in several different locations under the tree, the following results: SOLDIER STAND relocate STAND relocate STAND relocate STAND UNDER TREE. (Note that if STAND STAND STAND STAND is signed in the same location under the tree, this would be likely to be translated into English as a durative reduplication (Fischer, 1973): "The soldier (singular) stood under the tree for a long time." Additional examples of verbs which may incorporate number in their execution may be found in Bellugi and Fischer (1972).

A third way for the plural to be marked is for the signer to point with his or her index finger to the several locations under the tree where the soldiers are standing (see Figure 6): SOLDIER STAND THERE THERE THERE UNDER TREE.

Although the choice of pluralization strategy is partly a matter of taste, there are some constraints imposed by the manner in which signs are executed and by the real world. One would probably not sign BOOK GROUP; instead BOOK STACK would be more likely to be used, with STACK signed by indicating a vertical pile of them. Moreover, the real world may enter the picture in a vivid manner. Consider the sentence:

I left my books at home.

If the books were left at home stacked neatly on the table, the first solution, BOOK STACK, would serve. But if they were left scattered all over the house, BOOK THERE THERE THERE would probably be preferred. Other examples are not hard to imagine. The plural of CAR will depend on whether they are lined up on a highway or bunched up in the middle of a city. POTATO can be pluralized by adding the sack that holds them. MOSQUITO can be pluralized by imitating the amount of effort needed to swat them away.

Reduplication can also be used as a pluralization strategy when applied to the noun itself, although this does not seem to be appropriate in the case of SOLDIER. Some authorities report that the reduplicated SOLDIER SOLDIER SOLDIER should be translated into English as *army*. Even if that proves to be an assumption, namely, that a plural number of soldiers constitutes an army, additional problems stem from the fact that the sign SOLDIER is executed with both hands making contact with the body of the signer. One hand cannot be used to index plurality while the other makes the sign, a strategy that works very well for COWS, HORSES, and PIGS. Moreover, unless the signer shifts body position somewhat while SOLDIER SOLDIER SOLDIER are executed,

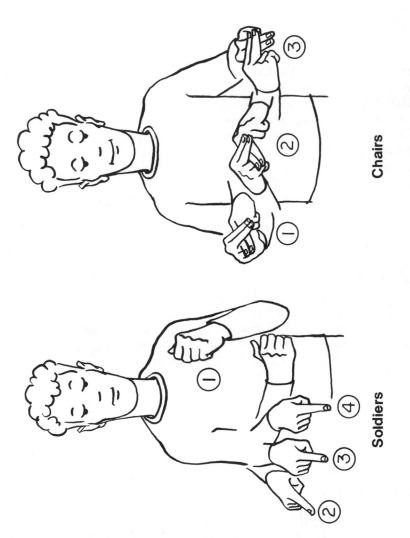

Figure 6.   SOLDIER may be pluralized by indexing several locations; CHAIR may be pluralized by reduplication.

the effect is to have all three signs executed in the same location. That seems to be a potentially ambiguous solution. But reduplication works very well for BOOK, CHAIR, PERSON, and a large number of other nouns. A list of nouns that can be pluralized by repetition has not yet been published. Meanwhile, students of ASL can test their "feel" for the language by making a judgment as to whether they think that specific nouns can be pluralized in this manner, and they can use their deaf acquaintances as informants to tell them whether their judgment conforms to deaf usage.

When nouns are pluralized by means of reduplication, additional information can be conveyed along with the repetition of the sign. For example, CHAIR CHAIR CHAIR can be lined up in a row or scattered aimlessly about (Figure 6 offers one alternative). DOG DOG DOG can be spaced close together near the signer or spaced far apart some distance away from the signer. In both cases, the structuring of the signed elements in neutral space incorporates information about the referents, namely, their spatial relationships to each other or to the signer.

Some restructuring has occcurred with reduplication for the pluralization of certain nouns. CHILDREN clearly is derived from a repetition of CHILD with constraints on the location and direction of movement. CITY has come from HOUSE, but with a shortening of the root sign. FOREST comes from TREE, but with a lateral movement required.

It must be kept in mind that pluralization strategies may be used in combination. For example, after adding GROUP to SOLDIER, the signer may still add THERE THERE THERE to add information about how the group was arranged, perhaps in a row at attention or perhaps scattered about. A signer may also let his eyes roam over the array of referents that are present in a plural number. Nonmanual stress markers may be added; for example, for "very many" the breath may be drawn in through pursed lips or clenched teeth as MANY MANY is executed (also see Chapter 20). The same cue added to FEW means "very few."

EXERCISES

Purpose

To give students practice in pluralizing nouns and in distinguishing plurals from singulars.

Instructions

The teacher should bring to class a number of sentences containing plural nouns and have the students: (1) indicate whether they understand the sentence as signed by the instructor to be a singular or a plural, or (2) execute the sentences in such a way that the plural marker is unambiguous. More than one pluralization strategy may be used where appropriate.

1. The cows were in the barn.
2. The cows were all over the pasture.
3. The cars were in the driveway.
4. The onions were on the counter.
5. I lost my books on the train.
6. I stacked the chairs in the closet.
7. I set up the chairs for the speech.
8. The chairs are not for sale.
9. The men were sitting on the bench.
10. The mice disappeared into a hole.

CHAPTER 6

COMPOUNDS

One of the ways in which languages may generate new vocabulary items is by a process of compounding. Two words may be joined together, typically with some measurable change in the pronunciation, with a different meaning resulting than would be inferred from the two words taken literally. Thus, a *bookworm* is not only a "worm that eats books" but also a "studious person," and a *lady killer* does not really go around committing homicide.

Compounds are also found in Sign (Klima and Bellugi, in press). Thus, THINK + REMAIN = REMEMBER, and LEARN + PERSON = STUDENT. Just as the phonology of spoken words may change when they are combined to form compounds (there is more separation and a different pattern of stress when one literally means a "key stone" and when one means a "keystone"), so also the execution of signs may be altered when they are combined into compounds. The sign THINK in THINK + REMAIN may no longer include a circular motion of the index finger on the forehead. The circle is reduced to a touch, or perhaps just a close approximation, and the touch may be made with the thumb of the right A hand instead of the index finger, in anticipation of the hand configuration to be used for REMAIN. The first part of the sign STUDENT may be raised only a short distance above the left palm instead of going all the way to the forehead. Sometimes the second part of the sign is affected by an elision instead of or in addition to the first. In BROTHER and SISTER the second portion, SAME, is likely to touch the index fingers together only once, not twice, or the right G hand may simply drop down on top of the left rather than align the index fingers side by side. Speed of execution of one or both elements is likely to be increased. This restructuring of the signs when they are compounded can be taken as internal evidence that a compound has been formed (Klima and Bellugi, in press). External evidence can be derived from the meaning that is assigned to the end product. If it is a compound, the meaning will be different, sometimes very different, from the meaning of the component signs that are used to form the compound.

Compounds typically pose no particular problems for students of Sign. As a matter of fact, many of them are learned from vocabulary lists as if they were simply another sign. But it helps to know that compounding is a feature of Sign, since new compounds are likely to continue to be formed as the language rises to meet additional challenges to its existing lexicon.

A special problem arises, however, when English compounds are translated literally into Sign. A compound is defined as a term whose meaning is something different from the literal meaning of the elements combined to form the compound. When translating from English to Sign, it is the meaning that must be rendered into Sign. The fact that a particular meaning was coded in English by means of a compound does not mean that it would be coded as a compound in ASL. In fact, even if it were, it is unlikely that the ASL compound would be comprised of the same elements as the English. A literal translation of the elements of an English compound into ASL is likely to result in ASL nonsense. EAT + CITY and SAVE + WAY are likely to be met by a frown unless the context makes it plain that we are referring to the Food Town or Safeway chains of grocery stores. Translators will often have to resort to paraphrases or neologisms to capture the meaning of some English compounds. For example, the English term "home made" should, perhaps, be translated into ASL as MAKE MYSELF, and "grownups" can be translated ADULTS (TALL TALL TALL with alternating left and right hands).

Although it does not seem that a great deal of time needs to be spent on the matter, students should, perhaps, be given some opportunity to see a list of compounds and to reflect upon their literal versus their actual meaning. The exercise below may serve that function. Meanwhile, the presence of compounds in ASL and their conformity to specific linguistic rules constitute additional evidence that ASL is a language, that it is not dependent on a spoken language for its internal organization, and that its grammar is accessible to linguistic analysis.

EXERCISES

Purpose

To acquaint students with some compounds and with the need to translate their meaning independently of the literal meaning of their component signs.

Instructions

Sign the following compounds and ask the students to give both a literal and an actual meaning.

1. THINK + REMAIN
2. BOY + SAME
3. FARM + person marker
4. THINK + GOAL
5. MONEY + WOW
6. BOY + BABY
7. KING + OVER
8. LEARN + person marker
9. FEMALE + MARRY
10. THINK + SAME

CHAPTER 7

FINGERSPELLING

It is recommended that students be introduced to the handshapes required for fingerspelling in a gradual way as the handshapes appear in signs. At least it should be made clear that fingerspelling should not be learned merely to avoid having to learn a larger sign vocabulary (Ingram, 1977).

Fingerspelling has become so well integrated into ASL usage that some fingerspelling configurations have taken on some of the characteristics of a sign (Battison, 1976, 1977). A movement such as a twist of the wrist has been added to some terms (j-o-b), and some of the letters have partially dropped out of others (w-h-a-t- $\rightarrow$ w-t). Still others sometimes involve a bilateral (two-handed) execution (n-o) or reduplication (n-o, n-o, n-o) to mean an emphatic "no." At least one example makes use of three types of restructuring—bilateral execution, reduplication, and a change in orientation: d-o, d-o, d-o means "What do you want to do?" Fingerspelled loan words constitute an important aspect of ASL usage that students need to master, and there has been considerable restructuring as these English words were borrowed by ASL (Battison, 1976).

A second use of fingerspelling is to add emphasis or rhetorical effect. Under some circumstances, the most emphatic way to say "no!" is to fingerspell it very deliberately, n-o. When one fingerspells for emphasis, the hand may be held out at arm's length, or both hands may be used at once. The hand doing the fingerspelling may be held closer to the receiver's face than is ordinarily polite (see Figure 7). The motion from one letter to the next may be made in a more abrupt and jerky manner than is customary, and the rate of fingerspelling may be slowed.

Finally, fingerspelling may be used simply to include English vocabulary items in a manual system. All societies that are in contact with one another seem to have a tendency to borrow each other's vocabulary under certain circumstances. Thus, we have *savoir faire* from French, *Gesundheit* from German, and *Sputnik* from Russian. That ASL should borrow from English is hardly surprising. Perhaps if English terms were not so readily available, the deaf community would have developed new signs, additional compounds, or an idiomatic paraphrase to refer to some of the things that they now customarily fingerspell, such

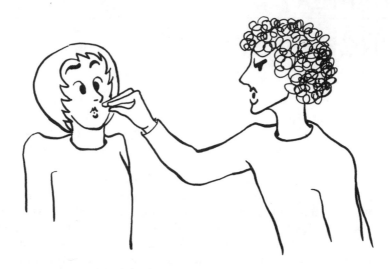

Figure 7. Spelling close to the receiver's face adds emphasis to the message.

as the brand names of merchandise, the months of the year, and many proper names. Unpublished data from a word/sign association test administered in 1976 to Gallaudet College students reveal that nouns were far more likely to elicit a fingerspelled association than were verbs and adjectives. This was the case regardless of whether the stimulus item was signed or fingerspelled. Apparently fingerspelling is well established among some users of Sign as a strategy for nominal refer- encing.

When fingerspelling, students should be urged to: 1) relax; 2) make no unnecessary movements of the arm or hand; 3) spell as rhy- thmically, not as rapidly, as possible; and 4) hold the hand in a com- fortable, neutral position in front of the right shoulder (Babbini, 1974; Fant, 1964; Guillory, 1966). They should be cautioned *not* to spell the letters aloud as they fingerspell them. If they say anything at all, it should be the word that they are spelling, not the letters that make it up, and they should say the word as they fingerspell it, not before or after- ward.

There is a rule in fingerspelling about doubling letters that students should know about (Madsen, 1972). When a letter is made by a touch (d, f, k, etc.), doubling is effected by touching twice. When there is no contact made (l, u, w), a slight forward or lateral movement is made to double the letter.

Some people pause between words, but the separation made by deaf persons when they fingerspell whole sentences is all but imperceptible to the non-native signer.

Fingerspelling exercises should not require students to fingerspell words or messages that would not be likely to be fingerspelled by deaf persons in the ordinary course of a conversation in ASL. The exercises should be confined to items that are likely to be fingerspelled.

EXERCISES

Purpose
To give students practice in sending and receiving fingerspelling.

Instructions
Spell the following sentences to students at a reasonable rate of speed. Do not fingerspell words for which there are common signs available. Do not slow down to a snail's pace when fingerspelling to students. Get them accustomed right from the start to an acceptable rate of fingerspelling.

1. Hemingway lived in Key West, Florida.
2. The A. G. Bell Association is in Washington, D.C.
3. St. Louis is in Missouri.
4. Philodendron is beautiful.
5. Bowling Green, Ohio, was named after Bowling Green, Kentucky.

Make up additional sentences using proper names well known to the students. Use some of the sentences to practice receptive skills and others to give students practice in executing fingerspelling.

Alternative Exercises

1. Write the names of each of the 50 states on index cards. Shuffle them and deal them out to students. Let them work in pairs spelling to each other one state at a time.
2. Do the same with names of famous people, brand names of merchandise, and names of cities.

CHAPTER 8

INCORPORATION

In Chapter 5 on pluralization, it was noted that the size of the sign GROUP could simultaneously say something about the size of the group. For example, a very large group of soldiers could be indicated by greatly enlarging the size of the sign GROUP. Moreover, it was pointed out that when reduplication was used as a pluralization strategy, location was incorporated in the pluralization. In the example given in Chapter 5, reduplication of the verb STAND had the effect of indicating where some soldiers were standing relative to each other. In another example, reduplication of the noun CHAIR had the same effect of incorporating location. Figure 6 in that chapter illustrates both of these examples.

Incorporation is a frequently occurring phenomenon in ASL, and some understanding of what it is and how it works would appear to be rather important for students and teachers of the language. The problem is complicated by the fact that the term is sometimes used in a slightly different sense that it is used for the balance of this discussion. Woodward (1974a) has coined the term *negative incorporation* to refer to a grammatical construction which is found associated with a small number of signs in ASL. It is characterized by a turning of the palm or hand away from the body "with an outward twisting movement of the moving hand(s) from the place where the sign is made" (Woodward 1974a). The effect is to negate the sign just executed. Examples of this usage are BAD (derived from GOOD), DON'T-LIKE (derived from LIKE), DON'T-WANT (derived from WANT), and DON'T-KNOW (derived from KNOW). This usage is well documented as a feature of ASL. The only question is whether it is a clear example of incorporation.

One way to think about incorporation is to see it as any rule-governed modification of the execution of a specifiable group of signs that has the effect of contributing additional predictable semantic content. In that case, the usage of negative incorporation, described above, should perhaps be allowed, as should incorporation of gender in the sign COUSIN (the TAB of the sign incorporates gender information). But this is probably too broad a definition, since it would have to accommodate also the manner in which nouns and verbs are distinguished in ASL (Supalla and Newport, 1976, 1978). This is an issue which the linguists will eventually have to resolve. Meanwhile, for the purpose of

clarifying matters somewhat, this discussion is limited to the presentation of examples from a variety of types of incorporation and to some
exercises which give students an opportunity to gain some experience
with this feature of ASL. It is based largely on the appendix which Susan
Fischer contributed to a more comprehensive article on Sign by Bellugi
and Fischer (1972).

Fischer lists four types of incorporation: 1) incorporation of location,   2) incorporation of number,   3) incorporation of manner, and 4)
incorporation of size and shape. These are not mutually exclusive
categories. For example, take the assignment to express in Sign the
following English sentence:

> The three men circled around toward my right
> and advanced slowly toward me on my right side.

In ASL one might represent the three men with the right 3 hand extended some distance from the body. The "circle to the right" could be
indicated by moving the hand around to the right and following it with
eyes. Then the hand could be brought slowly toward the signer's body to
indicate that the three persons were slowly approaching from that direction. Thus, we have incorporation of number in the DEZ of the sign and
incorporation of location and manner in the SIG of the sign.

Examples of incorporation of location are easy to find in ASL because spatial organization is such a pervasive feature (see Chapter 13).
A large number of verbs (but not all verbs) are modified in execution so
as to conform to the spatial organization that is implied by the spatial
frame of reference used by the signer (see also Edge and Herrmann,
1977). Among the verbs that can be modified in this way are the following: ADVISE, APPROACH, BORROW ("lend"), BOTHER, BRING,
COME (GO), COPY, FINGERSPELL, GIVE, HATE, INTRODUCE,
LEAVE ("abandon"), LEAVE ("depart"), LOOK, PAY ATTENTION,
QUESTION, READ, SHOW, and TELL.

If location can be incorporated into verbs, so can direction.
LOOK-UP, LOOK-DOWN, LOOK-AROUND, LOOK-BACK are clear
examples. Direction of movement can also be incorporated, as in JUMP-
UP, GO-AROUND, PULL-OFF-THE-ROAD, PARRALLEL-PARK, etc.

A discussion of incorporation of number in ASL would not be
complete without reference to the ease with which dual number is
indicated, a capacity lacked by English. The basic strategy for coding a
dual, on which there are many variations, is to sign one-handed signs
with both hands in tandem. Thus the sign SIT executed simultaneously
with both hooked V hands can mean that two people sat side by side.

Two raised index fingers moved in brief arcs toward the signer can mean that two people approached side by side. Two airplanes can be depicted flying in a wing-to-wing formation. The use of one hand to represent one person while the other hand represents another probably underlies the formation of a group of signs which have typically been considered to be independent lexical items but which may, in fact, involve incorporation of number and location as an essential feature, namely, FOLLOW, ACCOMPANY, AVOID, and ASSOCIATE. One member of that same group of signs, CHASE, would, according to this interpretation, involve incorporation of number, location, and manner.

Incorporation of manner is an adverbial function, affecting verbs and adjectives. Thus, to use two of Fischer's examples (Bellugi and Fischer, 1972), BEGIN signed very slowly means to "begin slowly," and FAMOUS signed in an enlarged manner means "very famous."

Size and shape are not the only descriptors that can be incorporated as nouns are signed. Weight, temperature, and even odor can be incorporated into signs. For a translation of the English sentence, "He picked up the dead fish and threw it in the trash," it is difficult to imagine signing PICKED-UP without some deference for the qualities of the object, and the sign FISH is likely to be removed as far as possible from the signer's body.

In role taking for direct discourse (see Chapter 19) the relative size of the various speakers may be incorporated in the execution of the signed statements. Deaf children describing referents in a communication task (Hoemann, 1972) incorporated size and shape in their one-sign executions BIG-CIRCLE and SMALL-SQUARE. Some verbs seem to invite incorporation of descriptors along with the incorporation of their objects (OPEN, THROW, GRASP, etc.). Without knowing what it is that is being opened, thrown, or grasped, it is hard to imagine how the verb would be signed.

Incorporation presents special problems for Sign to English translation, since the incorporated feature may have to be inferred by the translator on the basis of somewhat ambiguous cues (how big must the sign BIG be for it to become "very big"?) and since exact English equivalents of incorporation of location and direction are clearly lacking. For a general discussion of some of the issues raised by translation into and out of Sign, see Tweney (in press) and Tweney and Hoemann (1976).

EXERCISES

(1) Purpose

To give students practice in recognizing the information incorporated in signs.

Instructions

The instructor should sign the following items using incorporation of location, number, manner, and descriptors. Students should translate the executions into English.

1. LOOK-AT ME
2. JUMP-DOWN
3. BIG BRIDGE
4. VERY GOOD
5. TINY KEY
6. VERY SICK
7. PUNT THE FOOTBALL
8. SWAT THE FLY
9. SHOOT A RIFLE

(2) Purpose

To give students practice in modifying signs appropriately so as to incorporate additional information.

Instructions

Have students translate the following English sentences into Sign. Assist them with vocabulary if necessary.

1. I found a big ball in the street.
2. I looked up and saw many airplanes.
3. I parked the car under the tree.
4. That man is very famous.
5. The soup tasted awful.
6. I walked slowly toward the house.
7. The water ran all over the floor.
8. I waited for a long, long time.
9. My mother made me a big cake for my birthday.

CHAPTER 9

EMPHASIS AND STRESS

Of course, ASL has adjectives like BIG, STRONG, HEAVY, and FAMOUS, and it has adverbs like VERY and TRULY. But the English noun phrase, "A very big house," can be depicted by means of a variety of strategies in ASL that serve the same function as the English adverb *very*.

Some of these strategies involve variations on the sign for BIG. Ordinarily the two hooked L hands are drawn apart in front of the body. Some of the flourishes that can be attached for the sake of emphasis are: 1) lead with the right hand, follow with the left, and then shake both L hands in their extended positions; 2) start both hooked L hands outward and upward in a sweeping arc, and then bring them both downward sharply, ending in an abrupt stop; 3) bring the two hooked L hands outward in alternating circular movements, moving further out with each circular motion, until the two L hands are appropriately separated; and 4) bring the two L hands apart with alternating, sharply angular, zig-zag motions instead of circular motions. Any flourish attached to the execution of the sign for BIG adds stress to the adjectives. The flourish functions as an adverb. All of these flourishes are examples of incorporation of manner as described in the previous chapter.

A second set of strategies for adding stress to the statement, "a big house," is to exaggerate the size of the sign for house. Thus, the one gesture, all by itself, can mean "a very large house" (see Figure 8). Along with the exaggerated size, one can slow down the motion of the execution. Slowly executing an enlarged sign HOUSE incorporates both the adjective and the adverb in the modifications of the execution. This is an example of the incorporation of manner and size. It may be noted that the execution illustrated in Figure 8 violates the limits which ordinarily govern the sign space permitted for signs. Such a violation, all by itself, is likely to carry special significance for a signed statement. In this case, the effect is to add emphasis.

Another set of strategies involves facial cues that accompany the execution of BIG. Sucking in the breath through pursed lips or clenched teeth, puffing out the cheeks, or opening wide the eyes and mouth all have the effect of adding stress to the adjective. Both facial expression and body stance contribute to the emphasis attached to the sign DUMB-

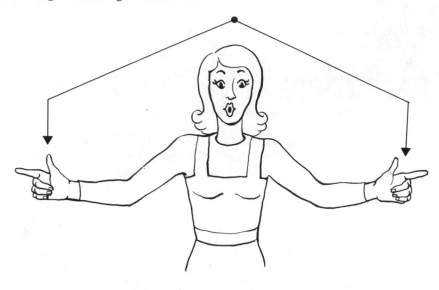

Figure 8.   An exaggerated sign for HOUSE incorporates both manner and size in one sign: "a very big house."

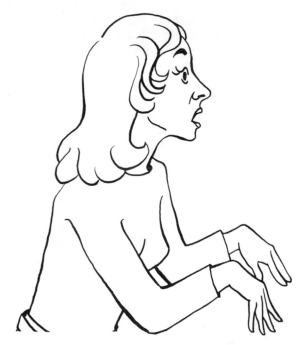

Figure 9.   The facial expression and body stance contribute to the meaning of DUMB-FOUNDED.

FOUNDED (Figure 9). These strategies are somewhat analogous to the contribution made to a spoken statement by the tone of voice. By prolonging the word "big" and by using a rising inflection, the spoken statement, "a big house," can also take on the meaning of "a very big house."

Finally, the signer can wait with the stress markers until the signs BIG HOUSE have been executed, and then a variety of "comments" can be added. The signer may add a shake of the head as if in disbelief at the size of the house. A hands-on-hip stance may accompany the head-shaking. Or the signer may add the sign for *wow*, shaking the right 5 hand at waist level. The wide-eyed, open-mouthed astonishment that was mentioned as possibly accompanying the sign for BIG may also be delayed until after the signs BIG HOUSE have been executed. In each of these latter instances, the stress is added by letting the receiver observe the effect that the BIG HOUSE has on the signer. This same strategy could serve equally well for other intensified adjectives: PRETTY GIRL, EXPENSIVE CAR, etc.

There are at least four strategies, then, for adding stress to the adjective BIG to translate the English "a very big house": 1) add a flourish to the sign BIG, 2) modify the execution of the sign HOUSE,   3) add a facial cue or other nonmanual stress signal, and   4) add an affective display after the signs have been executed. (For a previous discussion of features of stress in ASL, see Covington, 1973b.)

It should be added that these strategies are not used in isolation, but are ordinarily used in rich combinations of features that co-occur in ASL (Baker, 1976a, 1976b; Friedman, 1976). A flourish on BIG can be accompanied by puffed cheeks and followed by an astonished stare. Some special modification of the facial expression is likely to always be present when an adjective is intensified. Both the increased number and the mutual consistency of the stress markers that are added to a statement in ASL contribute to the redundancy that makes the statement easier to understand.

EXERCISES

Purpose

To give students practice in adding stress markers to a variety of adjectives and nouns.

Instructions

Let each student propose one or more solutions to the following adverb-adjective-noun combinations. The teacher should supply the necessary vocabulary.

1. A very nice day
2. A very pretty girl
3. A very loud noise
4. A very small dog
5. A very big ship
6. A very dirty boy
7. A very funny story
8. A very expensive car
9. A very sour lemon
10. A very strong man

CHAPTER 10

NATURAL EXPRESSIVE GESTURES

Very young deaf children exhibit the same emotional responses to things that frustrate or delight them as do children with normal hearing. An angry, stubborn.child is an angry, stubborn child, and looks like one, regardless whether he or she is deaf or hearing (see Figure 10). But

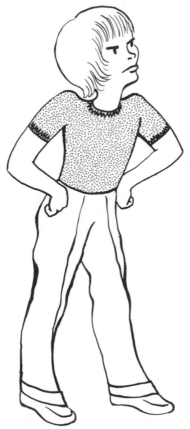

Figure 10.   Semantic content can be communicated nonlinguistically; an angry, stubborn child looks angry and stubborn.

there is a difference, and the difference is one that may be important for language acquisition. As hearing children grow older, they need to rely less and less on a display of emotion that the receiver must interpret. Instead, by the time they are four to six years old, hearing children are able to articulate their feelings and their wishes by means of spoken language. They no longer need to cultivate effective means of communicating information in a visual-gestural system. Deaf children never completely replace their visual system of communication with a different one. They continue to make use of a visible display of feelings and meanings as a part of their system of communication. Consequently, what one might call "natural, expressive gestures" can be said to play an important role in deaf children's communicative behavior.

But linguists get nervous when linguistic and nonlinguistic behaviors are not carefully distinguished from one another. In the case of deaf children's use of natural gestures, their concerns would appear to be well founded.

First of all, deaf children of deaf parents are likely to acquire linguistic competence in ASL from a very young age. This complicates an analysis of the role that natural gestures may play in their communicative acts, since expressions that would be considered "natural" or "expressive" in some sense when used by hearing children may be influenced in subtle ways by the manual language system that young deaf children are acquiring from their deaf parents.

Even when they are deprived of adult models of ASL and have only each other to help them master a visual language, deaf children may begin to modify natural expressive gestures in unique and systematic ways (Goldin-Meadow, in press; Goldin-Meadow and Feldman, 1975, 1977). A "natural gesture" that is part of a complex visual code or that has been systematically influenced by the linguistic context in which it occurs is, somehow, no longer "natural," not if it can be shown that the constraints governing its articulation are the same as those found throughout ASL usage. At least it is not safe to assume that identical events are taking place when an inarticulate hearing child exudes anger and hostility and when an enraged deaf child displays an appropriate combination of facial and body cues.

Evidence is lacking that deaf persons are more adept at displaying their emotions than are hearing persons. Certainly there are enormous individual differences, and the distributions are overlapping. Undoubtedly, some hearing persons are more adept at expressing their feelings naturally with gestures and with body language than many deaf people. But there is no denying that deaf people have a life-time of experience to support their use of visual means to communicate information about their feelings. And in ASL there is the interesting possibility of expressing the semantic content of a message manually and, at the same time, to indicate by means of facial and body cues how one feels about it. Unlike speech, where some of these cues are visual and some are auditory, ASL presents both the message and the subjective, editorial comment all in the same visual channel. The distinction between a facial cue incorporating manner and a facial cue signaling an editorial comment may lie in the temporal patterning of the facial expression relative to the signed statement (Liddell, 1977a). To indicate in sign, "I am angry," the same angry facial expression would probably span the entire statement. To indicate in sign, "I was surprised at how angry I was," might be indicated by changing the facial expression from one of anger to one of surprise as the sentence is executed.

In a spoken language, cues that assist the receiver in inferring the speaker's intent are often presented at least in part in the speaker's tone of voice. Sarcasm, pleading, joking, unwilling assent, incredulity, total agreement, or deliberate falsification can be signaled by the tone of voice at the same time that supposedly factual information is being given audibly. The ability to pick up these cues about how a message is to be understood constitutes part of what is included in sociolinguistic competence in a language. Such ability is not conferred automatically; it must be learned. This means that one must be a member of a particular culture or society to know how to distinguish and interpret these cues.

In the case of visual displays of emotion, it would seem that all members of a society, deaf and hearing, would share the same set of differentiated responses. In that case hearing persons should have no special difficulty interpreting the natural gestures which deaf people add to their manual communications. For the most part, this seems to be true. Emotions which differ greatly from each other are associated with expressive movements and appearances that also differ greatly. But ASL is not a "universal language" (Battison and Jordan, 1976; Jordan and Battison, 1976), and there are grounds for suspecting that hearing persons are not privy to all of the nuances and shades of meaning that deaf people code in their facial expressions, body postures, tension in certain muscles, and movements. Reliance on speech may reduce hearing people's sensitivity to nonverbal communication, and in our culture we are trained to restrain our expression of feelings and emotions. Deaf people, on the other hand, may have fewer problems with letting their feelings show, and they may learn to read one another's moods, attitudes, and reactions with a great deal of accuracy. Their manual system of communicating can take for granted that this ability is a part of the competence that characterizes native users of ASL.

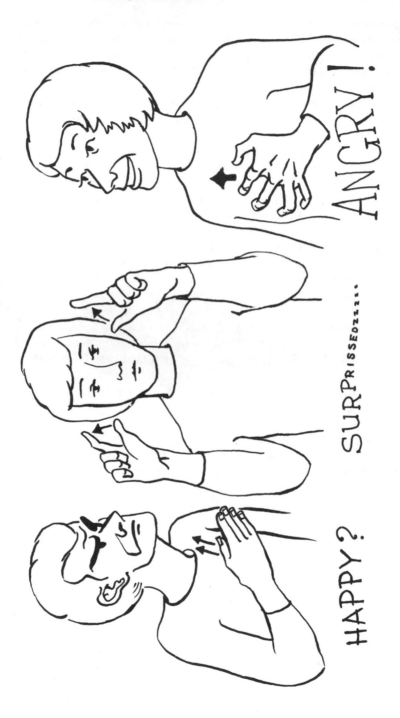

Figure 11. Facial expressions with inappropriate affect would be inappropriate in a spoken language; they might be ungrammatical in a sign language.

In fact, it may even be the case that facial expressions that are reliably understood by deaf people as having a certain meaning (e.g., a stress marker corresponding to the English word *very*) might be misconstrued by a hearing person who lacks experience with ASL as meaning something else (e.g., anger or hostility).

In any case, the same information that is coded both visually and auditorially by speakers of English when they say things like "I am surprised," or "I am angry," must be coded entirely in a visual mode by speakers of ASL. No one says, "I am angry," with a completely flat, emotionless expression. By the same token, no one should sign, I ANGRY in ASL without letting the anger show in the body stance, the facial expression, and even in the vigor with which the signs are executed. What is inappropriate behavior in a spoken language may be an ungrammatical behavior in a sign language. (See Figure 11). Students of ASL should be given practice at recognizing and using appropriate facial and body cues for expressing one's emotional state. The following exercises may help.

EXERCISES

(1) Purpose

To give students practice in reading and sending appropriate facial and body cues.

Instructions

Write the following "messages" on index cards, shuffle them, and deal them out to small groups of students in the class. Have the students take turns trying to express nonverbally the message on their card. The other students should try to guess what it is.

Set one: fear, surprise, anger, relief, boredom, grief.

Set two: resentment, jealousy, anxiety, suspicion, melancholy, disgust.

Set three: annoyed, sorry, peeved, relaxed, happy, spacy.

Set four: Don't do that, shut up, I like you, say something, let me alone, Huh?, Let's get acquainted, What happened?, I'm sorry, Help me.

(2) Purpose

To give students practice exhibiting a facial expression, body stance, and mode of execution that is appropriate for a given statement.

Instructions

The teacher should sign the following sentences with an inappropriate expression. Let the students indicate what is wrong with the statement as executed and correct it by adding an appropriate expression.

1. I was surprised (signal *bored*).
2. I was afraid (signal *angry*).
3. I was disappointed (signal *surprised*).
4. I was angry (signal *afraid*).
5. I was happy (signal *cross*).

CHAPTER 11

PANTOMIME

Deaf persons often weave Sign and pantomime together along with natural expressive gestures into a single system of visual communication that draws on a variety of resources to achieve its goals. Developmentally, deaf children become proficient in Sign and in pantomime concurrently. They learn these elements of visual communication not as separate entities but as complementary resources.

Not all pantomime executions are to be considered as a part of American Sign Language. If a particular execution is understood by the general public, and if no special training or experience with the language is needed to understand the meaning of the exeuction, then there is no particular reason for thinking that this is an example of a manual language production. On the other hand, if the only persons who can understand an execution are those who have had an opportunity to develop linguistic and communicative competence in a manual language, then it is appropriate to consider the production to be an example of Sign rather than pantomime.

When mature deaf persons resort to pantomime as a communicative strategy, it is likely that elements of American Sign Language will be found along with adept imitations, and a linguistic analysis of pantomime in American Sign Language may uncover a variety of subtle differences between the pantomime used by deaf persons and the pantomime generated by a professional mime. Although nonspecialists may view the pantomime of a professional mime and the mimetic productions of a user of ASL as similar, these behaviors may be viewed very differently by linguists. To the extent that the mimetic productions of deaf persons are rule governed, embedded in ASL, and not fully understood by those who do not understand ASL, they are qualitatively different from the pantomime productions of the performing artist.

Students of ASL need to deal with pantomime as an important feature of visual communication. They should be on the lookout to detect the subtle differences that might be found between pantomime as a part of ASL and pantomime in our performing arts or parlor games. The manner in which deaf persons make use of pantomime as they communicate may sometimes reveal interesting and important aspects of their personalities. In any case, some action sequences are much easier to

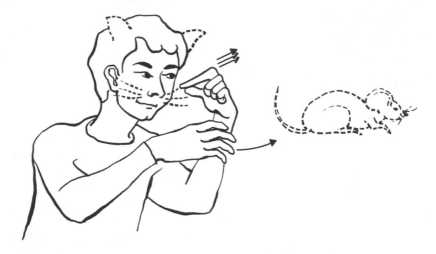

Figure 12.   A signer may even personify an animal stalking its prey.

portray in narrative order by acting them out than they are to explain "verbally" in a spoken or manual system.

Students should be advised that they have a great deal of latitude when they use pantomime to communicate a message. For example, the signer may personify an animal stalking its prey (Figure 12) or devote considerably more time and attention to detail in a narrative than is ordinarily given in a communication. Even the element of time is used creatively rather than realistically. It is not the case that real time and the time it takes to pantomime an action coincide exactly, although they may. Pantomime may stretch time out for clarity or telescope it for dramatic effect. The important thing to keep in mind is that pantomime is drama, and the sender must put on a show that is both clear and interesting.

Second, pantomime is not restricted to the set of locations and movements that are structural features of ASL. The hand configurations tend to be those that are naturally assumed, as when holding an object or participating in an activity. Much more space can be exploited for the action, and the sender's body will serve as a symbol far more frequently and extensively than in formal signing.

Third, whereas Sign tends to derive its vocabulary from a single aspect of a referent, such as the beak of a bird or the roof and walls of a house, pantomime is likely to abstract several features and use all of them for the sake of clarity. The bird may be given an eye and a tail and then cling to a branch as the signer's head imitates the jerky movements of a songbird. The house may be given windows, a door, a sidewalk, and a man walking up to the door and pushing the bell. There is no hurry.

The more features that can be added skillfully, the more interesting and informative is the result.

The following exercise is designed to give students practice in making use of pantomime to enliven their ASL productions.

EXERCISES

Purpose

To clarify the distinction between Sign and pantomime and to give students practice in the use of pantomime as an alternative means of translating or expressing meaning.

Instructions

Students should sign each of the following in conventional ASL and then provide a pantomime translation. They may make additions or changes to each other's proposed pantomime versions.

1. I opened the letter and read it.
2. I took a bite out of the sandwich and found a bone in it.
3. I reached for some change in my pocket and found that I had a hole in it.
4. I looked both ways and then darted across the street.
5. I inspected my bleary-eyed face in the mirror.
6. After I wound and set my new watch, I put it on my wrist and admired it.
7. I hooked my (golf) shot off to the left and into the woods.

The instructor may also make up a deck of index cards, each card containing a specific action sequence to be pantomimed. They may include a wide variety of challenges, e.g., a drunk walking down a flight of stairs, a cat stalking a mouse, a tired horse plodding along a road, a squirrel hiding a nut, a spider spinning a web, etc. With patience and ingenuity a teacher can collect a couple hundred items of this nature. They can be used either at the beginning of class as an ice breaker or during the middle as a welcome diversion or change of pace.

STRUCTURE IN ASL PHRASES AND CLAUSES

Knowing a language means much more than knowing its vocabulary. It means being able to construct novel, meaningful, well formed sentences and being able to recognize sentences that are ungrammatical or ambiguous.

Knowing ASL means much more than knowing a large number of signs. It means being able to understand and to express meaningful statements in ASL that exploit the full range of strategies available in the language for effective communication.

This is an ambitious goal for a hearing person who wishes to learn ASL as a second language. But this is the kind of knowledge of the language enjoyed by native speakers, people who have learned the language spontaneously from their childhood.

Something needs to be said about the extent to which deaf persons are bilingual in English and Sign (Charrow and Fletcher, 1973; Charrow and Wilbur, 1975; Kannapell, 1974; Markowicz and Woodward, in press). With few exceptions deaf persons know both Sign and English to a greater or lesser degree of competence. It is probably safe to assume that most deaf children who attended a residential school for the deaf are more proficient in Sign than English. Sign serves as their first language, especially among their peers, and English is used with members of the larger society. Deaf persons may also modify their Sign productions when communicating with a hearing person. Out of deference to the likelihood that the hearing person is not proficient in Sign, the deaf person may use what is known popularly as signed English, a product of the pidginization or creolization of Sign in the United States (Fischer, 1976; Woodward, 1973c); Woodward and Markowicz, in press).

But not all deaf persons are native users of ASL. Many of them had hearing parents who did not know or use ASL with them when they were very young. It was not until they went to school and met other deaf children, some of whom knew ASL, that some deaf persons began to learn the language. Some deaf persons may have had no opportunity to learn ASL from their peers until they were young adults (Padden and Markowicz, 1976). The only deaf persons who can be said to have had a completely natural opportunity to learn ASL as native users are those whose parents were deaf and used ASL at home (Cicourel and Boese, 1972). It has been discovered that deaf children tend to develop a manual system of communication among themselves even when they are deprived of models in ASL in their environments (Goldin-Meadow, in press; Goldin-Meadow and Feldman, 1975, 1977). (See Kuschel, 1973, for a commentary on the sign language used by the only deaf person on a Polynesian island.) It might be argued that this qualifies the children observed by Goldin-Meadow and Feldman as native users if their subsequent development includes assimilation into the deaf linguistic community. But the fact is that we do not know what effects on language competence might occur as a function of early deprivation from adult models. This is why researchers studying ASL prefer to use deaf children of deaf parents as informants.

To become as fluent as possible in ASL, students need to take note of the features of ASL which provide structure for phrases and clauses, features which organize signs into meaningful sentences. Sign language structure at this level is grammatical structure, and the grammar of ASL is the set of rules and principles that govern permissible usage and that make possible unambiguous inferences regarding the meaning of statements made in ASL.

In English, word order plays a prominent role in structuring sentences. Sign order in ASL is not as tightly constrained as is word order in English. Tervoort's (1968) example, YOU ME DOWNTOWN MOVIE FUN exaggerates the amount of freedom of order that is found in ASL. Although his discussion agrees with earlier commentaries (Fusfeld, 1958), it has been shown that order constraints do exist in ASL (Hoemann and Florian, 1976). Fischer (1975) has discussed the possibility that ASL sign order has changed over time as a result of influence from English. The subject of sign order in ASL is somewhat controversial at this time. An extensive discussion of the issues at stake can be found in Wilbur (in press).

One of the most pervasive structuring features of ASL is spatial organization. This is not surprising, considering that ASL depends on a visual channel. This second section of this volume begins with Chapter 12 and a rudimentary description of the signing space that is available for the ordinary use of the language. One of the differences between ASL and pantomime is that pantomime does not recognize the boundaries on space for signing that act as constraints on ASL usage. Like most rules, there are exceptions, and the situations that allow a signer in ASL to alter or to ignore the normal constraints on sign space are also very informative.

Chapter 13 deals specifically with some of the meaningful and grammatical distinctions that are accomplished in ASL by means of spatial organization (Bellugi and Fischer, 1972; Edge and Herrmann, 1977; Ellenberger and Steyaert, 1976; Friedman, 1977b; Hoffmeister, 1977; Kegl and Wilbur, 1976; Wilbur, in press). Pronominal reference, referent description, direct-indirect object distinctions, agent-patient differentiation, and the coordination or subordination of clauses are all candidates for spatial organization of ASL messages. An attempt is made in Chapter 13 to link spatial organization as a grammatical strategy to psychological and developmental aspects of language use.

Temporal relations and durations are also organized in ASL at least in part by means of spatial arrangements (Frishberg, 1975; Frishberg and Gough, 1973). But the speed with which a sign is executed may also affect the meaning in a reliable manner, and the facial expression may contribute confirming or supplemental information. Chapter 14 deals with the way in which ASL marks tenses and the way it codes temporal concepts.

Once it has been verified that spatial organization, manner (speed and force) of execution, and facial expression are all implicated in the structure of ASL sentences, specific kinds of sentences can be examined for information on how their meaning is coded reliably in ASL. Chapter 15 compares and contrasts indicative, interrogative, and imperative sentences (statements, questions, and commands) in order to obtain information regarding the role or roles played by the various resources that the signer has available for coding meaning.

Chapter 16 examines conditional sentences and the variety of strategies available for coding real and unreal conditions and their consequences (Baker and Padden, 1976, in press; Hoemann, 1976).

Chapter 17 is devoted to juncture markers, the cues that tell the receiver where one phrase or clause stops and where another begins. Nonmanual features of ASL are also important for marking junctures, and this chapter provides another opportunity to stress their importance.

Chapter 18 discusses eye gaze, a feature of ASL that has linguistic, sociolinguistic, and even psycholinguistic aspects. Through eye gaze (or lack of it) ASL users control conversations, make pronominal references, enhance their referent descriptions or verb presentations, add stress to individual words and to portions of narratives, and participate in the activities that relate them and the imaginary world of referents that they organize around themselves spatially (Baker, 1976a, 1976b, 1977; Baker and Padden, 1976, in press).

Chapter 19 discusses role taking, which has a specific utility for dealing with direct discourse but which also has a more general function in ASL for dealing with narrative as a literary form.

Chapter 20 of this section deals with an aspect of signing on which there are, as yet, no published data, namely, the relation between breathing behavior and signing. While breathing does not affect signing as directly as it does speaking, inhaling, exhaling, and holding the breath clearly have the potential of affecting the meaning of a sign or a signed sentence. Chapter 20 includes some possible examples.

The last chapter, Chapter 21, is devoted to song and poetry in Sign. It mentions internal and external sources of poetic structure (Klima and Bellugi, 1975b, 1976) and identifies some individuals and groups who are currently making a contribution to ASL literature and art as poets, playwright, and performing artists.

As in the case of the first section, these 10 chapters are not intended to serve as an exhaustive treatment of the grammatical structure of ASL. The topics included in the second section were selected for their value in introducing students and teachers to aspects of ASL that heretofore have not been given adequate treatment in a "Sign Class" and that need to be mastered if the student is to come anywhere close to becoming a fluent user of the language.

CHAPTER 12

SIGN SPACE

Signs tend to be executed in a certain definable region relative to the signer's body (Friedman, 1975, 1977a). Only a small number of signs are executed above the head (SUN, SKY) or below the waist (TROUSERS, DOG). Most signs are executed between the waist and a point just above the forehead and within easy reach of the signer, left and right. Moreover, the signs are not executed far out in front of the body, but within a comfortable distance, with bent elbows. Conformity to this sign space produces accommodations to the structural features of signs that were discussed in Chapter 1 of the first section. For example, a mime might communicate "picking a flower" to the audience by bending over and plucking an imaginary flower from the ground. A deaf user of ASL will use his or her upturned left palm as the TAB for the sign, and the right F hand will pluck the imaginary flower from the left palm.

The basis for a sign space is probably largely physiologic. Signs are executed in the region that is most comfortable for the signer. Constraints based on human physiology affect the *articulation* of signs. This is the case also for other sign languages, e.g., the sign language of the Trappist Monks (Barakat, 1969, 1975).

Siple (in press) has observed that even within the sign space there are differences between the signs executed near the face, where peripheral vision is likely to be most acute, and signs executed in the outer regions of the sign space. Signs made on the face and upper body display much finer distinctions in handshape and location than signs made outside this region. Signs executed within this focal region are likely to manifest only small differences from one another and to be executed with relatively small movements. Signs made in the peripheral areas of the sign space are likely to be symmetric, two-handed signs differing greatly from one another. Constraints based on visual acuity affect the *perceptibility* of signs.

Individual differences will affect the sign space. A large person with long arms will encompass more space with signing than will a person with short arms. An outgoing, exhuberant person will extend his or her sign space much more than will a shy, withdrawn person.

Other influences on sign space are interesting and important. A signer before a large audience will enlarge his or her sign space so as to be more readily understood, much like a speaker will raise his or her voice to be heard, while a person engaged in an intimate or private conversation will constrict the sign space to conform to the mood of the situation. These accommodations indicate that it is not merely the convenience or ease of the signer that determines the space of signs but also the signer's awareness of the needs of the receiver(s).

Violations of the normal constraints imposed by the sign space may function as meaningful cues to the speaker's intent. Like other nonverbal cues, they function as a signal for how the speaker expects the message to be understood. For example, a signer who extends the arms farther forward than is normal so as to "straight-arm" the receiver has added a noticeable amount of emphasis, perhaps even hostility, to the message. This is especially the case when the extended arm winds up closer to the receiver's face than is considered polite.

Another example of a violation of sign space may occur when a person wants to address a third party briefly without interrupting conversation with a signer. Let's assume that a mother wants to discipline a child who is behaving in an unruly manner. Without breaking eye contact with the signer, the mother may extend her right arm toward the child, even if the child is behind her back, and sign FINISH. Executing the sign outside of the sign space serves as a cue that the sign is directed toward some audience other than the person with whom the mother is conversing.

Displacement of a sign from its normal location to a point outside the sign space may be an effective rhetorical device for setting an item or an action off for special treatment. The sentence I GO CHICAGO NO signed with CHICAGO positioned somewhere off in "left field" instead of in front of the right shoulder, where it ought to be, can set the stage for signing, NO, directly at the displaced CHICAGO. The net effect is a strong statement, translated into English as *I am definitely not going to Chicago*. Using the same strategy, CHRISTMAS may be signed so far out in front of the body that the effect is to indicate that it is too far in the future even to contemplate. In Figure 8 the sign HOUSE is depicted with an execution that enlarges the sign so much that it lies outside the sign space. The effect is to incorporate the adverb and adjective *very large* in the execution. Thus HOUSE + a violation of the sign space = "a very large house."

To take one more example of a sign space violation, if a man leaves his right arm draped over the arm of a sofa and signs to someone sitting next to him in a very casual, abbreviated manner, with his signs barely discernible and perhaps not even understandable to a stranger who might be looking on, the failure of the signer to accommodate to the sign space is a mark of intimacy, a clear announcement that the signer and the receiver are so close to each other that each is able to understand even the most casual ASL utterance. On the other hand, a person who wants to be very formal and reserved in ASL discourse with a receiver will conform quite exactly to the constraints generally imposed on the sign space.

Language use permits a variety of speaking (or signing) styles, ranging from very casual and intimate styles of speaking to very formal, stilted styles of speaking. Stokoe (1971) has discussed the various ways in which signing styles may differ along this same dimension. Germane to this discussion on sign space, it appears that a formal style is far more likely than the intimate style to accommodate to the constraints of the sign space. This has important implications for some forms of manual communication. Persons using signed English as their preferred language modality or persons who are communicating by means of the simultaneous method, speaking and signing at the same time, are also far more likely to box their signs into a small space front and center at their chest. They may even avoid moving signs closer to their face so that they do not obscure their lip movements. Such behaviors may make it very difficult to achieve an intimate rapport with an audience. Indeed, a person using the simultaneous method may be perceived by a deaf receiver to be a very reserved, formal, perhaps even unfriendly person. This is highly speculative, of course, but the relation between speaking styles and receiver perceptions is clear enough to warrant some attention to the effect of accommodating to a formal style of signing. Institutions with a heavy committment to the use of the simultaneous method have begun research on various aspects of its use (Caccamise and Blasdell, 1977; Caccamise and Johnson, in press). Attention to the effect that such a communicative mode has on receivers' perceptions of speakers would appear warranted.

EXERCISES

Purpose

To acquaint students of ASL with the variety of cues that may be associated with violations of the sign space.

Instructions

The instructor may sign each of the following statements with the associated nuance (indicated in parentheses), and students may be invited to guess at the probable intent.

1. FINISH (Signed far above the head with a cheerful facial expression as if to say, "I thought I would never get it done")
2. YOU LIVE FAR (Extending the sign FAR outside the sign space as if to imply that it is too far to be acceptable)
3. I WILL BUY (Extending the sign BUY farther forward than the sign space allows to imply great eagerness to buy something)
4. FINISH (Signed far off to the right with a smug facial expression as if to imply relief that something is done)
5. KNOW AGO (With AGO or PAST signed far back over the shoulder as if to imply, "I knew that a long time ago")

CHAPTER 13

SPATIAL ORGANIZATION

Spatial organization is used in ASL for such a wide variety of purposes and with such a diversity of creative and individual applications that a comprehensive treatment is all but impossible. The best that teachers of ASL can do at this time is to introduce spatial organization with a variety of examples, point out some of its more important functions, and trust that the students' further experiences with ASL will continue to enhance their appreciation for the central, organizing role that the appropriate use of space can serve.

To illustrate the effective use of spatial organization in ASL, this chapter cites pronominal reference, referent descriptions, direct-indirect object distinctions, agent-patient distinctions, and coordinate and subordinate phrases and clauses.

To refer to someone or something that is physically present, one needs only to point to it, and this is the case whether one is using a manual or a spoken language system. In fact, in ASL, if the referent is physically present, an arbitrary point would not be assigned for later reference; the signer would merely point to the referent. But languages also need an unambiguous means of referring to persons or things that are absent (anaphoric reference). This is the function ordinarily served by pronouns in English. *He* can refer to a man not in sight, and *it* can refer to something that has never been seen at all.

The organization of referents and potential referents in space around the signer allows for a similar capability in ASL. Once a referent has been included in the spatial organization that is constructed for a narrative and has, therefore, acquired a location on this imaginary stage, pointing to a location for an imaginary referent has the same effect as pointing to the referent itself, as if the referent were physically present. This simple description, however, does not do justice to the complexity of the strategy. If the referent is mobile, the direction of the point may shift as the referent changes location during the action portrayed. This indicates that it is not really a location per se that is the object of the pointing sign but an imaginary object at that location. Moreover, the pronoun may be incorporated in the handshape as the verb is executed. For example, consider the statement (in English), *Put it* (the can) *on the shelf.* In ASL the C handshape would grasp an imaginary can so that the verb would include a reference to what it was that was being shelved. Thus, the spatial organization that makes pro-nominal referencing possible in the first place also allows the signer to participate in the world of make believe objects and to alter signing behavior to incorporate size, shape, weight, etc.

Referent descriptions are enhanced by spatial organization whenever the physical relation of features of the referent or referents are salient. For example, if I wished to describe the location of my office on the BGSU campus, I would say in English, "It is on the second floor of the Psychology Building, down the hallway to the left from the elevator, the fourth room on the right." In ASL I could first identify PSYCHOLOGY BUILDING, then point upward and sign SECOND FLOOR, sign GO-UP, LEFT, FIRST, SECOND, THIRD, FOURTH, pause, and then point to the location marked as FOURTH. As the ordinal numerals FIRST, SECOND, THIRD, and FOURTH are executed, the hand could move away from the body toward the left as if proceeding down the hallway. Then, when the final pointing sign is executed to the fourth room, it could be aimed toward the right rather than toward the left to indicate that the fourth room on the right is intended.

Or consider the assignment given the man who must explain to his wife where in the parking lot he parked the family car. He might begin by signing STORE and pointing directly downward in front of his chest. Then he could indicate by means of an inverted index finger (GO) which direction from the store entrance his wife would have to go to find the car, whether to the right, straight ahead, or to the left. Notice that the verb GO has been modified to fit the spatial organization imposed on the scene, with the result that the motion of the verb corresponds to the desired direction of movement. Then, with the side of his palm chopping off rows he could count how far from the store the car was to be found. After the required number of rows had been counted off, the signer, again using his index finger, could indicate approximately how far into the row the wife had to go in order to find the car. The final message might be translated in English, *From the store go four rows to the right and then walk toward the opposite side of the lot, about half the distance to the street. You will find the car in that area.*

A second important function of spatial organization in ASL is the unambiguous distinction of direct and indirect objects (Bode, 1974; Friedman, 1975). Direct-indirect object distinctions in English are made clear by means of word order. "I showed the robber the policeman" means something quite different from "I showed the policeman the robber." In ASL, the policeman and the robber would first be assigned specific locations, probably on the left and the right of the signer. Then the direction of the verb SHOW will indicate who was shown to whom.

Agent-patient distinctions may also be made in ASL by means of spatial organization of the sentence. Consider the example (in English), *Paul met John on the street, and he hit him.* In English, this sentence is ambiguous; to make it unambiguous the statement would have to repeat one of the nouns in the second clause. In ASL it would not be unusual for one of the principals, perhaps John, to be assigned a location in front of the signer. J-o-h-n THERE, ON STREET. To make it plain that it was Paul who met John and not the other way around, the sign MEET could be executed in such a manner that the left hand remained stationary, representing John, and the right hand, representing Paul, could be moved forward from the body (P-a-u-l MEET). Then the sign HIT could be executed in the same direction to mean that Paul hit John, or it could be executed directly toward the signer's face to indicate that John hit Paul. The direction of movement of the verb incorporates the agent-patient distinction (Bellugi and Fischer, 1972).

Spatial organization also facilitates the separation of phrases and clauses from each other. Suppose we wanted to say that in a snow storm it makes no difference whether you are stuck at home or in some other house, you just have to wait it out. The two phrases, YOUR HOUSE and OTHER HOUSE, can be assigned side by side locations in front of the body at the same elevation. The sign SAME can be executed across both of them or the sign MAKES-NO-DIFFERENCE can be signed midway between them, and then the conclusion can be added, MUST WAIT. Now let's imagine that we want to say something quite different, namely, that to be stuck at home is better than being stuck in some other house. Now STUCK HOME can be signed off to the right at a slightly elevated position, and STUCK OTHER HOUSE can be assigned a lower, debased position off to the left. The lower position of the phrase on the left compared to the right is sufficient to assign it a less attractive status.

To ask someone if he or she wants coffee or tea, COFFEE can be signed off to the left, and TEA can be signed off to the right. WHICH can then be signed in such a way that its sign space encompasses both of them. Notice that the use of the interrogative WHICH eliminates a need for explicit use of the conjunction OR. Similarly, when phrases or clauses are ordered parallel to one another in space, the conjunction AND can be assumed to be incorporated in the spatial organization of the sentence; the sign AND is unnecessary.

Points that are being enumerated in a speech (first, second, third, etc.) can be arranged spatially left to right, so that the transition from one location to another signals that the speaker is moving on to the next point. Staying in the same location indicates that the signer is still discussing the same point. Other devices for marking transitions between points in a speech that involve space in some way are a change in head position, a shift of body stance, or a change in handedness for signing.

A subordinated spatial location relative to the normal sign space that has been used can also set off a subordinate clause from the main clause or set off a parenthetical expression from the main drift of the statement. A lowering of the location may be accompanied by a reduction in sign space used for the subordinated clause or for the parenthetical expression.

Clearly, if grammar is the glue that holds sentences together, then spatial organization plays a major role in the grammar of ASL. By means of spatial organization, signs are related to each other (TABLE + LOOK UNDER = "Look under the table"), and to the signer (LOOK (toward) ME = "Look at me"; GIVE (toward) ME = "Give it to me"). Such relationships between signs forge them together into phrases and clauses.

The centrality of spatial organization for ASL grammar has important implications for manual language systems which forego spatial organization in order to achieve some conformity to English grammar. Such a wedding of Sign and English may yield a result that is unsatisfactory from the standpoint of either language system. The various manual sign systems (Anthony, 1971; Bornstein, Saulnier, and Hamilton, 1976; Coats, 1948; Gustason, Pfetzing, and Zawolkow, 1972; Mossel, 1956-1957) relinquish one of the most pervasive strategies found in ASL for organizing semantic content into a coherent linguistic statement, namely, spatial organization, and they have no analogue for vocal inflection and intonation for making important grammatical or syntactic distinctions. Such a "least common denominator" of two dissimilar languages leaves only a subset of the strategies that would otherwise be available for coding information. Thus, manual sign systems sacrifice the tonal inflection of spoken languages and the spatial organization of sign languages. The result may be increased ambiguity in the constructed messages. (For a variety of opinions on the educational implications of signed English systems, see Cokely and Gawlik, 1973, 1974; Cornett, 1967; Markowicz, 1976; Mayberry, 1978; Moores, 1973, 1977; and Wilbur, in press.)

Cognitive theories of psychology assign responsibility for the spatial organization found in ASL to the phenomenologic perspective of the signer. The construction of ASL sentences presupposes a prior cognitive construction of a physical situation, a temporal frame of reference, a real world context for the information that is to be transmitted. If it is a specific location that gives the information its setting, the sender projects that location around him-or herself in space, and all of the props and characters that are included in that projection are immediately available as things that could be referenced. In communicating that setting to another person, the sender does not need to delineate every detail, but may specify only so much as is needed to provide structure for the message. Later, the signer may index a specific location by pointing to it, and this will serve as a pronominal reference to whatever is imagined to be at that location. Eye gaze (see Chapter 18) may also serve as a pronominal reference, and sign verbs may incorporate a pronominal reference to a direct or indirect object by modifying the hand configuration or the direction of the hand movement. These strategies also provide some of the internal structure for sign language sentences. Especially interesting (and evidence that the sender's phenomenologic perspective is the source of spatial structure) is that the sender's eye gaze may roam over the imaginary contents of the setting that he or she is creating as if he or she were surveying the field, deciding what to discuss first. Clearly, there may be mental contact between the sender and the imaginary world that is the subject matter of his or her discourse.

At the same time, the spatial organization that is designated by the sender must be recognized and understood by the receiver. This may require some rather sophisticated role taking on the part of the receiver of ASL. Receivers must be able to relate their understanding of a message to the staging developed by the signer. They must be able to imagine the characters and props projected by the signer in their appropriate locations on the stage. Moreover, receivers must mentally transform the sender's spatial frame of reference in order to understand positions and movements relative to their own vantage point.

This is no small assignment. From the perspective of Piaget's theory, concrete operatory thinking is required to support such a complex coordination of perspectives. Pre-school deaf children are limited in the extent to which they can construct a complex, imaginary spatial network of agents and patients. But they make an interesting and effective accommodation to their cognitive immaturity. Since they lack a mental structure that can construct a complex coordination of perspectives, they make use of the real, physical situation in which they find themselves to impose spatial structure on their ASL productions. Thus, when they wish to refer to an absent person or object, they may point to a location where the referent is customarily found. To refer to "teacher" when the teacher is out of the room, they may point to the blackboard where the teacher is ordinarily located. To refer to "mother" or "home," a young residential school pupil may arch the right arm and point to a far distant place. (Adult signers retain this strategy for referring to distant places or times.)

This implies, of course, that the language capacity of deaf children is a function of their cognitive capacity rather than the other way around. For far too long it has been believed that deaf children cannot think unless they "have" a language. On the contrary, unless deaf children can think, and unless by means of thought they can create a spatial frame of reference for their language, their linguistic productions will reflect their cognitive limitations.

With development, deaf children tend to organize their messages spatially. Deaf children in the primary department of a state residential school for the deaf were recently given four weeks of training in referential communication. One of the tasks in which they were given supervised practice required them to describe a picture of three objects in such a way that a peer receiver could identify it from other pictures in the array. All of the pictures contained the same objects; the only way they could be distinguished from one another was by way of their spatial arrangement or their physical relationship to one another. For example, the target picture presented a milk carton with an apple behind it and a cup and saucer on the right. The other pictures had the apple and cup located in a different manner relative to the milk carton (see Figure 13). Four of the 36 children included in the study showed some inclination on the pretest to organize their message spatially. Following training, 18, or half of the pupils, organized their message spatially for at least some of the trials in the posttest. Most of these children were only eight to ten years old. Their pretest performances were rather unsatisfactory. But their improvement with only minimal training was impressive, and many of them readily mastered strategies for coding meaning that are part of the manual system of communicating used by deaf adults, including spatial organization. Many of them also made use of spatial ordering to identify items by means of their position in a series, for example, the "third largest circle" or the "second smallest line." It may be the case that the training was especially effective because it allowed the pupils to model for each other the strategies that they discovered to be successful in the context of peer to peer communicating.

Students of ASL must learn in a short course what deaf children have a lifetime to learn to do; to integrate their perceptual and linguistic systems so as to yield symbolic representations of their world as they see it, imagine it, and understand it. The following exercises are designed to introduce students to the use of an imaginary stage or a phenomenologic field to impose structure on ASL productions. Receptive skills are stressed first.

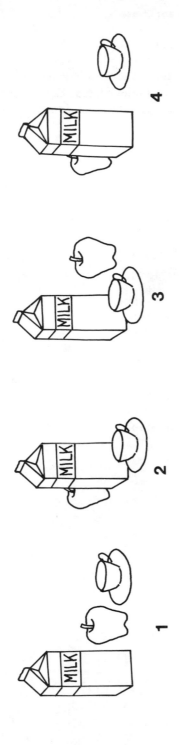

Figure 13. To distinguish the fourth picture in an array from the other items in a referential description task, deaf children learned to organize their description spatially: APPLE (point away from chest), MILK (point close to chest), CUP (move hands over to the right).

EXERCISES

(1) Purpose

To introduce students to spatial organization as a strategy for structuring ASL productions and to recognize the meaning implied by spatial relations between signs.

Instructions

The teacher should execute the following in ASL using spatial relations to organize the information. Students should be urged to discuss the import of spatial references and to imitate brief segments of each narrative.

1. (Position a robber on the left.) Robber there. (Position a policeman on the right.) Policeman there. Wave to the policeman as if to attract his attention and then point repeatedly and emphatically in the direction of the robber.

2. When I first entered the room, I could see that the person living there had expensive tastes. On the wall to my right was a fine painting with a special light focused on it from the ceiling. On the floor was a thick carpet and nice, soft chairs spaced comfortably apart. A bear-skin rug was on the left side of the room in front of the fireplace. An ornate light fixture hung from the ceiling, and directly opposite from where I was standing, French doors opened out on the garden.

(2) Purpose

To give students practice in organizing information spatially.

Instructions

Have the students describe the room they are sitting in, including the furnishings and fixtures. Have them mark off in their imaginations a rectangle in front of them, and have them use that rectangle to arrange the contents of the room.

CHAPTER 14

TEMPORAL DURATIONS AND RELATIONS

There are basic gestures in ASL for the *past* (palm over the right shoulder), *present* (hands dropped down to a full stop in front of the waist), and *future* (hand moved forward from the right shoulder). These temporal regions are associated with the respective spatial domains located over the shoulder, in front of the body, and forward from the

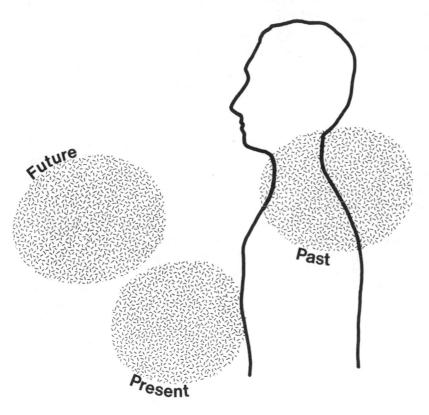

Figure 14.   The past, present, and future are represented, in part, by means of a spatial frame of reference.

shoulder (see Figure 14). Once a temporal frame of reference has been established, e.g., the past, it remains in effect until changed, and all the subsequent verbs are construed as in the past until and unless the temporal frame of reference is changed. All other temporal references are construed as relative to the basic frame of reference that prevails for the entire sequence.

Within the spatial domain that is used for temporal references there are a variety of mechanisms for expressing various durations of time and relations between temporally spaced events that require some discussion (Friedman, 1975; Frishberg, 1975; Frishberg and Gough, 1973).

The basic forward or backward movement is also found in the signs TOMORROW and YESTERDAY, LATER and PREVIOUSLY, POST-PONE and MOVE-UP (in time). NEXT-YEAR and LAST-YEAR, NEXT-WEEK and LAST-WEEK.

Proximity (the recent past or the imminent future) is indicated by contracting the body into a tight stance (shoulders hunched, head tilted, mouth pulled by tightening the muscles of the right cheek) and by miniaturizing the sign (Liddell, 1977a). Thus, NEXT-YEAR signed in a contracted stance implies that this is a very short time from now, and WHILE-AGO signed in a contracted stance implies that this was only a short while ago.

In contrast, a loose body stance (head tilted back, muscles relaxed, and mouth sagging open) and an enlargement of the sign denotes the opposite. NEXT-YEAR signed with a loose body stance implies that this is a long way off, and WHILE-AGO signed in the same manner means that this was quite some time ago.

Lest it appear that these features of ASL are tightly constrained and uniform among all signers, it must be added that there are many ways of displaying a contracted or a loose body stance. Exactly how one signals immediacy versus remoteness by means of body stance may be a matter of taste, training, or personality. Not everyone signs the remote future with the mouth sagging open. But one may; and until all of the component features of various body stances have been catalogued and correlated with one another and their respective meaning or meanings have been identified, we must be content with contrasts that are somewhat crude in measurement and, sometimes, in manner.

Moreover, there are ways of indicating the remote future other than by relaxing the body stance. Pursed lips, squinted eyes, and an exaggerated forward movement of the right hand may also be used to mark the remote future (see Figure 15).

The speed with which a sign is executed also affects the meaning. TOMORROW signed at normal speed means just that. Slowed down and

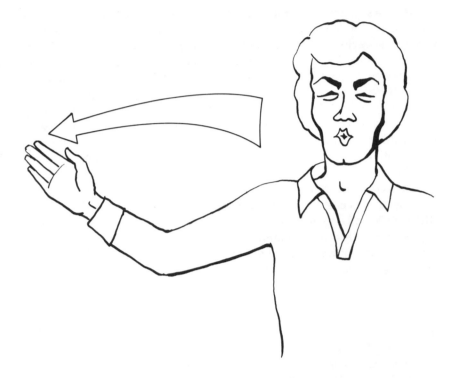

Figure 15.   The remote future may be indicated by means of pursed lips, squinted eyes, and an exaggerated forward movement of the right hand.

signed with a forward lean and frown, it may mean "tomorrow, not some other time." Speeded up and signed with pinched lips and a squint it may mean "tomorrow for sure." Certain signs (DAY, WEEK), when signed very slowly, become durative ("all day," "all week").

The basic citation form of temporal signs may also be subject to complex modulations. The number of weeks or years in the past or future can be indicated by the right hand configuration at the same time as the sign is executed. Thus we have NEXT-WEEK, TWO-WEEKS-FROM-NOW, THREE-WEEKS-FROM-NOW, LAST-WEEK, TWO-WEEKS-AGO, THREE-WEEKS-AGO, NEXT-YEAR, TWO-YEARS FROM-NOW, THREE-YEARS-FROM-NOW, LAST-YEAR, TWO-YEARS-AGO, THREE-YEARS-AGO. Again, a subjective impression as to whether these intervals are considered to be a short time or a long time can be marked simultaneously by the contracted versus loose constellation of facial and body cues described previously.

Another modulation that can be imposed directly on the citation form of WEEK, YEAR, MONTH, and other signs is to repeat the sign three or more times. Linguists call this "reduplication." Thus, YEAR + YEAR + YEAR = "every year," WEEK + WEEK + WEEK = "every week," MONTH + MONTH + MONTH = "every month," TOMORROW + TOMORROW + TOMORROW = "every day," ONCE + ONCE + ONCE = "sometimes." Here, too, other cues play an important role. Facial and body cues, especially the rapidity with which the reduplicated sign is executed, can make the difference between ONCE-IN-A-WHILE ("occasionally, relatively frequently") and ONCE-IN-A-WHILE ("rarely, almost never") (Fischer, 1973).

A slow, reduplicated, circular motion may be imposed on either a verb or an adjective to denote continuous action. For example, SICK SICK SICK signed in a circular motion toward the forehead, and preceded or followed by a sign for the past (AGO), means "I was sick all the time," or, "I was sick for a long time." WAIT WAIT WAIT with a similar circular execution means (in English) "I waited for a long time." (For a discussion of this and other verb modulations in ASL, see Pedersen, 1977.) The effect is not greatly different from what one gets in English from "I waited and waited and waited." But in ASL, in addition to the reduplication there is a circular modulation that is generalizable to a number of verbs and adjectives.

Fast reduplication tends to connote habitual or repeated action (Fischer, 1973). Thus, I GO GO GO STORE means "I went to the store again and again and again." Similarly, I FORGET FORGET FORGET means "I keep forgetting," or "I am a forgetful person."

The spatial domain that is invoked to represent past, present, and future may use the body or parts of the body as a frame of reference. An imaginary line drawn down the right side of the body allows movements forward from the body or cheek to take on a future connotation and movements backward from that line to take on a past connotation. Another line runs horizontally past the front of the body, so that movements forward across that line are future (POSTPONE) and movements backward are past (MOVE-UP-IN-TIME). Dropping the hands vertically in a full stop on the line means "now." A third line runs down the left palm when it is held with the fingers pointing upward. This is the same left hand configuration that is used for HOUR, MINUTE, SECOND, and for one of the signs for *time*. The right hand or right index finger moves on the left palm in the same direction as the hour and minute hand on a clock. From this frame of reference on the left palm one can indicate "later, after a while" with a forward movement, and "while ago, previously" with a movement of the finger toward the signer's body.

These signs can be executed either on the left palm or on the right cheek with essentially the same fields of meaning.

Since space is continuous, it affords the user of sign language considerable latitude to carve it up in a variety of ways in order to convey subtle nuances of time (Coulter, 1977). As a matter of fact, the distant future can be indicated by moving the right hand a full arm's length forward, and the distant past can be indicated by moving the right palm farther back over the right shoulder than is comfortable. Additional flourishes can add further emphasis: 1)   the movement can be executed as a series of short movements, with each movement extending farther in the appropriate direction; 2)   air can be sucked in between pursed lips or between clenched teeth and the eyes may be squinted shut as the sign is slowly executed; 3)   the movement can be executed in an exaggerated arc, as if spanning a great deal of time in between; and 4)   the movement can be made with both hands alternately moving forward or backward in a circular motion to indicate the distant future or distant past, respectively.

Two signs require special treatment, FINISH and NOT-YET. Both refer to past action, but the first refers to action completed in the past while the second refers to action that has not yet occurred in the past. Examples of the first, FINISH, are found in great numbers in ASL usage, since it is a frequently used sign. I GO FINISH means "I have already gone" or "I went." I FINISH SEE means "I have already seen it." FINISH is frequently used as an imperative, meaning "Stop that!". Madsen (1972) has listed a number of examples of idiomatic usages associated with the sign FINISH.

The sign NOT-YET serves as a negation of completed action in the past. EAT NOT-YET means "I haven't eaten yet" and SEE NOT-YET means "I haven't seen it yet."

The student of ASL can hardly be expected to move easily into the complex set of strategies and the variety of modulations found in ASL for indicating temporal relations and durations. As a start, some practice with specific connotations is appropriate. As always, receptive skills should be stressed first.

EXERCISES

Purpose

To introduce students to the manner in which space is used to indicate time and to provide practice in translating specific nuances of ASL executions.

Instructions

The instructor signs each of the following, and students translate them into English.

1. A LONG TIME AGO
2. JUST A FEW SECONDS AGO
3. TWO YEARS FROM NOW
4. NOT NOW; TOMORROW
5. EVERY DAY
6. A LONG TIME FROM NOW
7. ONCE IN A WHILE
8. INFREQUENTLY (rarely)
9. A LITTLE WHILE AGO
10. LATER
11. LAST WEEK
12. EVERY MONTH

Depending on the sophistication of the students, this exercise could be expanded to include practice in inferring more subtle nuances of ASL usages regarding time. Some productive practice could also be given, especially with the addition of a numeral to a temporal sign (e.g., TWO WEEKS, THREE YEARS), reduplication (WEEK WEEK WEEK = "weekly"), the circular, durative modulation (WORK WORK WORK = "work for a long time"), etc.

CHAPTER 15

QUESTIONS, ANSWERS, AND COMMANDS

Interrogatives, indicatives, and imperatives are marked in ASL by a complex set of events that occur together with considerable consistency. Because the cues are consistent, there is very little ambiguity in ASL with regard to these matters. A native user of ASL knows quite well whether he or she is being asked a question, given an answer, or told what to do.

The best way to illustrate the differences that mark the executions of these various sentence forms is to take a few simple examples. Take the one-sign sentence, NOW.

If the question had been asked, "When should I do it?" the appropriate answer might be NOW. The hands would drop down to a stop just above waist height. The facial expression would display neither strong emotion nor an inquiring attitude. After the sentence had been completed, the hands and arms would drop back to a neutral position just above the waist or in some other relaxed position. This is the indicative mood, and the sentence is a declarative sentence.

Questions require very different treatment. Consider the question, "Should I do it now?" This can be translated with the single sign NOW, provided some other things are also happening. Eyebrows are arched. Eye contact with the receiver, although probable in the short declarative sentence NOW, is certain for the question, NOW? The hands are not relaxed and returned to a neutral position; instead, they are held in the final pose for a considerable period of time, almost as if they will stay there until an answer is forthcoming. There may be a slight forward lean of the body and a slight forward thrust of the head. These features are intensified if the question were, "Do you really mean now?" The location for the execution of the sign NOW may be slightly farther forward, a little closer to the receiver than in the case of the declarative statement, NOW. Again, if the nuance of the question is, "You don't mean now, do you?", the sign might be executed very close to the receiver's face. The execution of the sign is likely to be somewhat slower than for the declarative NOW.

For the imperative "Do it now," facial and body cues are altered considerably. The downward movement of this sign is much sharper, and the stop at the bottom is made more forcefully. The brows are likely to be lowered, as in a frown. The lips may be pinched tightly shut. The torso may lean slightly backwards so as to leave the body firmly planted in place. Alternatively, imperatives may also be signed with a forward lean, but it is assertive rather than inquiring. A downward sagging of the shoulders may accompany the downward movement of the sign. As before, emphasis may be added by: 1) executing the sign closer to the receiver,   2) exaggerating the facial features accompanying the sign, and   3) executing the sign in a different manner, in this case, more forcefully. In comparison with the executions of the declarative sentence, NOW, and the question, NOW?, the imperative, NOW!, is signed very quickly. Eye contact is also very probable with imperatives.

To summarize, interrogatives take longer. They require raised brows, eye contact, and a forward lean. And they hold the final pose. Imperatives are executed quickly. They require lowered brows and probably maintain eye contact. The body leans forward or stands firmly in place. Imperatives are signed more forcefully. They may also hold the final pose. The indicative is not marked by raised or lowered brows. The execution is neither prolonged nor quick and forceful. The body stance is a relaxed, upright position. Following the statement, the hands and arms are returned to a neutral position.

Of course, declarative sentences can also be keyed to provide clues to the speaker's intent. A very casual, off-hand execution, perhaps with only one hand and with a minimal downward movement may imply, "It is OK to do it now." A shrug preceding the execution makes that interpretation even more likely. Conversely, if the facial expression is a wide-eyed, enthusiastic show of pleasure, the effect is to add an exclamation point, "Oh yea! Do it now!"

To take another example with a somewhat longer sentence, one can either say, ask, or command, (in English):

I left the cat in the house.

Did you leave the cat in the house?

Leave the cat in the house.

Using the sign LEAVE that is sometimes glossed as "abandon," all three sentences can be signed with the same four signs: LEAVE CAT IN HOUSE. What marks them as different are the other things that are happening while and immediately after the signs are executed. For the declarative statement, the signs are executed at a moderate rate. Eyebrows are in a neutral position, neither raised nor lowered. Eye contact is not required, and it may be broken during the course of the statement, returning to make eye contact with the receiver only if some kind of response is expected. After the sentence is completed, the hands and arms return to a neutral position at rest.

For the question, the brows are raised, eye contact is made and sustained throughout the question, and the head and body may assume a forward lean. After the sign is executed, the hands and arms are not returned to a rest position, but are held in somewhat the same position or location that they found themselves when the sign for *house* was completed. The raised brows are also held beyond the time when the last sign is executed as if awaiting an answer.

For the imperative, the brows may be lowered. The eyes may be slightly squinted. The sign LEAVE will probably be executed more distinctly and more forcefully. The four signs may be executed staccato, with noticeable junctures between each sign. The entire sentence may be executed more quickly than the declarative sentence. Or, alternatively, the imperative may be signed with an exaggerated slowness, so that each sign has an opportunity to impress itself on the receiver's consciousness.

It should be added that the features described in this chapter are not as obvious to the novice student as they are to the native signer of ASL. The facial and body features that mark interrogatives and imperatives as distinct from the indicative and as different from each other will often be obscured by other nuances—such as exasperation, surprise, delight, or dismay—that use the same features and are simultaneously being marked by the speaker. Moreover, individual differences in personality and signing style will be reflected in the clarity with which some of these features are manifest in a particular situation. Teachers of ASL should first assist students in habitually taking note of what the facial and body features are doing so that they learn to take this information into account as they try to infer meaning from what is signed. Then, with experience, students may become more and more adept at interpreting subtle cues regarding the signer's intent at the same time they recognize whether a sentence is a question, an answer, or a command.

EXERCISE

(1) Purpose

To give students practice in interpreting whether a sentence is a question, an answer, or a command.

Instructions

Let the teacher sign the following "sentences" as questions, commands, and declarative statements (in a random order for each set), and have the students report whether the sentence is interrogative, imperative, or indicative.

1. Get money. Get Money? Get money!
2. You go? You go! You go.
3. Make cookies. Make cookies! Make cookies?
4. Find car! Find car? Find car.
5. Bring book. Bring book! Bring book?
6. Work hard tomorrow? Work hard tomorrow! Work hard tomorrow.
7. Send boy home? Send boy home! Send boy home.
8. Do better. Do better! Do better?
9. Show picture! Show picture? Show picture.
10. Write letter? Write letter. Write letter!

(2) Purpose

To give students practice in marking sentences appropriately for the indicative, imperative, and interrogative.

Instructions

Have the students execute each of these one-sign sentences as: 1) questions,   2) commands, and   3) declarative statements.

1. GO
2. PITY
3. COMPLAIN
4. WATCH
5. WAIT
6. WIN
7. FILL
8. SIGN-YOUR-NAME
9. DO
10. FLY (by plane)

CHAPTER 16

CONDITIONAL SENTENCES

English introduces conditional clauses with the particle *if*. Real conditions, those whose consequences will take place provided the condition is fulfillled, take the indicative mood:

> If I have the money, I will buy the car.

Unreal conditions, those whose conditions cannot be fulfilled and, therefore, whose consequences will not follow, take the subjunctive mood:

> If I had the money, I would buy the car.

In ASL there are two ways to introduce a conditional sentence. One is to make use of a particle equivalent to *if*, either by fingerspelling the English word or by using the sign listed in the Stokoe, Casterline, and Croneberg (1965, p. 58) dictionary. It is similar to JUDGE, but it uses less space. The other way to mark the condition is to sign it as if it were a question and to mark the consequence as a statement of fact. Along with the raised eyebrows for the questioning expression, the sender may hold direct eye contact with the receiver during the conditional clause so as to establish heightened rapport. For the consequence, the raised eyebrows are dropped abruptly, signaling the boundary between the clauses as well as the changed "tone of voice." The first sentence above, then, becomes:

> HAVE MONEY? BUY CAR.

But what if the condition is an unreal condition? ASL has no construction comparable to the subjunctive mood. How is an unreal condition marked in ASL? One way is for it to be made completely clear that the condition cannot be satisfied or that the consequence was never realized. Once it is made plain either that there is no money or that no car was bought, then the rest of the conditional sentence can be executed as before.

> HAVE MONEY NONE. HAVE MONEY? BUY CAR.

> BUY CAR NONE. HAVE MONEY? BUY CAR.

An alternative method of signing unreal conditions is to mark the negation with facial features while the condition is being expressed

(Baker and Padden, in press). If this is done successfully, the consequences will, of course, remain unfulfilled. For example, if HAVE MONEY is signed with lowered brows, a slight squint, and slightly pinched lips, the effect is to indicate that the statement is not to be construed as a statement of fact. Instead, the receiver is to infer that the signer does not have the money.

Of course, if the condition is contrary to a readily observable fact, then it is not so difficult for the receiver to infer that it is an unreal condition. If it is raining hard, and the signer says (again with lowered brows, squint, and pinched lips), NOT RAIN, GO-OUT, PLAY, it is quite clear that it is raining and that, therefore, the condition will not be fulfilled.

At the very beginning of a course in ASL, students should not be expected to produce well formed conditional sentences. But with a minimal vocabulary, they can be taught to recognize them. As students begin to shed some of their inhibitions about using facial expression and changes in body stance to communicate, they can be expected to mark conditional clauses of real conditions with a questioning facial expression and to mark conditional clauses of unreal conditions with a negating facial expression or with an overt statement of fact.

This strategy for dealing with conditions succeeds, in part, because of the close rapport that is ordinarily established between the sender and the receiver in ASL. Sign seems to have evolved primarily as a face to face langauge for close social communication. By means of signs (UNDERSTAND? YOU-KNOW?) and by means of facial cues senders may frequently request some indication that the receiver is following the gist of the message. The receiver may frequently nod or sign YES to indicate that the sender may proceed. Questions posed by the sender enhance the rapport between the sender and receiver. Thus, when the sender signs questioningly, RAIN TOMORROW?, the receiver can begin to speculate about the possible consequences of an affirmative answer to the question, "Will it rain tomorrow?" Then the sender supplies the answer to his or her own question by adding, STAY HOME ("I will stay home"). Or, with our earlier example, if the signer frowns and signs wistfully, HAVE MONEY, the receiver knows that the sender does not have the money or the sender would not have signed it that way. Consequently, the receiver can reliably infer that no car is going to be bought.

EXERCISES

(1) Purpose

To introduce students to an effective strategy for marking conditional sentences and to give them some practice in Sign to English translation.

Instructions

The instructor should supply the necessary vocabulary (bed, broke, eat, excuse, friends, hungry, lonesome, make, tired, work). The instructor should sign the following brief sentences, and students should translate them from Sign to English.

1. SICK? EXCUSE ("If you are sick, you may be excused.")
2. BROKE? WORK ("If you are broke, go get some work.")
3. LONESOME? MAKE FRIENDS ("If you are lonesome, make friends.")
4. HUNGRY? GO EAT ("If you are hungry, go eat.")
5. TIRED? GO BED ("If you are tired, go to bed.")

(2) Purpose

To give students practice in executing conditional sentences by using a questioning expression for the conditional clause and an assertion for the consequence.

Instructions

The instructor should execute the following sentences, and the students should attempt to imitate not only the signs but also the facial expression and body language of the instructor.

1. HAPPEN TEMPERATURE PLUNGE, WILL BEGIN SNOW.
2. RAIN DISAPPEAR, ALL DRY.
3. ME RULE, MAKE FINE.

The instructor can provide additional examples.

CHAPTER 17

JUNCTURE MARKERS

There are four clear types of juncture markers in ASL. They mark the boundaries between signs, signed phrases, and clauses, providing important sources of structure for ASL sentences. (Also see Covington, 1973a; Grosjean and Lane, 1976, 1977.)

The first is any kind of change in a facial expression, body posture, or body orientation that has been sustained for a period of time. For example, the narrative depicted in Figure 16 implies that changes in facial expression will separate the segments of the narrative appropriately. It should be noted that if a change in facial expression can indicate a juncture, then the sustained facial expression across a particular phrase or clause helps to relate the signs to each other that are included in the phrase or clause so bracketed.

The preceding chapter on conditional sentences has already introduced the notion of a change in facial expression or body posture as playing a role in the structure of a sentence. The juncture marker separating a conditional clause from its consequence is the change from the questioning to the assertive facial expression and body posture that occurs between the two clauses. This kind of juncture marker, then, is displayed not so much by something that one does but by something that one stops doing or that one does differently than before.

Second, pauses are used in ASL in much the same way as in English (Grosjean and Lane, 1976, 1977). A pause generally separates clauses, and shorter pauses separate phrases within clauses. Still shorter pauses may separate signs from each other. Eye blinks may frequently occur during such pauses (Baker, 1976a). These separations are more apparent when the rate of signing is slowed down (Grosjean and Lane, 1976, 1977). In rapid signing, only the pauses between major sentence segments may be marked clearly. However, it must be kept in mind that sophisticated users of ASL may detect pauses that beginning signers are unable to see.

A third juncture marker is a characteristic position or posture that may be assumed at the end of a clause or sentence. Statements of fact are followed by a relaxation of the arms and a neutral body stance. Questions are followed by a body stance characterized by an expectant pose and an inquiring facial expression, both of which indicate that the signer is awaiting a response. An exclamation, on the other hand, may

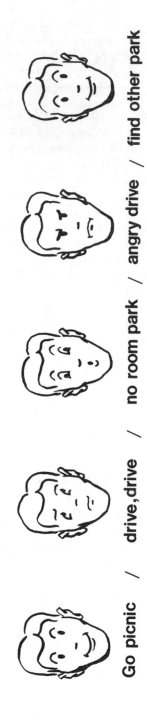

Go picnic / drive,drive / no room park / angry drive / find other park

Figure 16.   A sustained facial expression links the signs together as a phrase or clause; changes in facial expression mark the junctures between phrases and clauses.

be followed by an assertive nod of the head and a body stance that signals surprise, belligerence, or enthusiasm, depending on the circumstances. Such a body stance may be held for a brief duration following the message.

A fourth juncture marker is a change in location for the execution for a sign or a series of signs. For example, if one wished to make the point that during the day time one worked but at night had fun, the person might sign DAY WORK off to the left of center and then sign NIGHT FUN off to the right of center. The change in location would serve as a cue (but not the only one) that these are distinct clauses, separated by a clear juncture.

It should be apparent from this discussion that if students of ASL execute their signs deadpan without any change in the location or in the mood with which they sign them, it will be rather difficult to tell where one phrase ends and another begins. It would be very much like a monotone in a spoken language, with nothing to link the words together into longer units or to divide the entire sequence into its component parts. Interpreters who are signing a spoken address need to be especially careful to retain juncture markers in their interpretation. If they are having a hard time keeping up, they will be tempted to shorten the pauses between phrases and clauses and to make less frequent use of changes in location or facial expression. But this puts an added burden on the deaf audience to understand the ASL version of the presentation. Interpreters must take time to signal the beginning and the end of their ASL sentences by making appropriate use of markers that are available.

Juncture markers may appear in combinations. A change in location will require a brief pause between the executions, and a change in body orientation may be accompanied by a change in facial expression as well. Boundaries between phrases and clauses are marked quite clearly in ASL. There is ordinarily no doubt as to what goes with what.

EXERCISES

Purpose

To give students practice in recognizing the junctures between phrases and clauses and to make use of juncture markers to separate ASL sentences.

Instructions

Sign the following sentences to the students and have them indicate which signs should be understood as grouped in phrases. Then have the students sign the pairs of sentences and indicate the difference in meaning that each version implies.

1. RAIN-FALL/TOMMORROW MUST STAY HOME.
2. RAIN-FALL TOMORROW/MUST STAY HOME.
3. BUY CAR/NOW CAN VACATION.
4. BUY CAR NOW/CAN VACATION.
5. HAVE MONEY/MUCH FUN FUTURE.
6. HAVE MONEY MUCH/FUN FUTURE.
7. GO MOVIE INTERESTING/NEVER SEE BEFORE.
8. GO MOVIE/INTERESTING/NEVER SEE BEFORE.
9. MAKE COOKIES/FORGET SUGAR/TASTE TERRIBLE.
10. MAKE COOKIES FORGET SUGAR/TASTE/TERRIBLE

CHAPTER 18

EYE GAZE

Novice students of ASL have a marked tendency to watch the hands of the person who is speaking to them in Sign. It would probably be a good idea for teachers of ASL to discourage that practice right from the beginning, for two reasons. First, deaf people do not do it; native competence is characterized by a very different kind of looking behavior and gaze control, some aspects of which are important features of knowing and using ASL. Second, it reflects an inappropriate emphasis on what the hands are doing to the exclusion of some important events transpiring on the face. In any case, Siple (in press) has shown that Sign activity which takes place in the peripheral regions of the customary sign space is composed of signs that are larger, more redundant, and more discrepant from one another than the signs that take place near the face and upper chest region. Students who learn to look to the face of the signer, even maintaining a reasonable amount of eye contact, can trust that they are looking where most of the action is. They can also trust that Sign as a language has evolved to fit the human visual perceptual system that has to take it in.

Baker (1976a, 1976b, 1977), Padden (1976), and Baker and Padden (1976, in press) have identified several specialized uses associated with control over the direction of the gaze or line of vision while executing signs.

First, Sign requires very different strategies than are found in spoken languages for controlling the ebb and flow of a conversation. It is simply not possible in ASL to "shout someone down" or to interrupt someone merely by butting in louder. In fact, in ASL there is a very effective strategy available for keeping people from butting in at all; one must simply avoid looking at them. Children of deaf parents seem to learn at a very young age that they can avoid being disciplined by their parents by simply looking off to the side and by refusing to look the parent in the face. It is not uncommon under such circumstances for a parent to physically turn the child's head toward his or her own so as to be sure to have the child's attention.

How does one "interrupt" a signer engaged in a monologue? Baker (1977) advises that the receiver should wait until the signer happens to make eye contact at a juncture between clauses and then immediately do two things at once: 1) start signing, and 2) look away. Needless to say, native speakers of ASL know when they have been interrupted, and they may react just as predictably as people who are interrupted in a spoken language.

Baker (1976a, 1977) has estimated that the signer is looking away from the face of the receiver as much as half the time. One reason for this is that eye gaze assumes a number of linguistic functions in ASL, and these require looking somewhere else than at the receiver. Of course, when the signer wants to yield the floor to the receiver, eye contact will be established with the other person, who is given time to begin signing.

One of the linguistic functions of eye gaze is to serve, along with pointing, as a means of pronominal referencing. Once people or objects have been organized spatially relative to the signer, the signer can refer to one or another of these referents simply by directing a gaze toward the location of the imaginary referent. This is especially useful when both hands are tied up making the sign, so that a pointing response would interrupt the flow of the message. While signing CAR, for example, a glance or head nod or both in the direction of someone standing near or toward a location established for an individual serves the same purpose as pointing to the person or the location.

Baker (1976a) has suggested that a "secretive gaze" directed toward the inside shoulder may serve as a surreptitious pronominal reference in private conversation. Such references are made very quickly, generally without an accompanying head nod, since it is intended that the person to whom reference is made will not be aware that someone is talking about them. This strategy does not seem to be unique to ASL: sidelong glances have served a useful function both for actors and actresses in the movies and for social comments carried out in the real world.

Baker (1976a, 1976b) believes that some signs are more likely than others to be accompanied by a specific kind of eye gaze. Some examples mentioned by Baker are IMAGINE, ALL, GROW-UP, QUOTE, SEARCH, and MOUNTAIN. In some cases it may be the iconic nature of the referent that invites (imaginary) visual inspection (MOUNTAIN). In other cases the execution of the sign may elicit a participation in the activity that is appropriate at the time (SEARCH, IMAGINE). It seems that when a signer chooses to act out a narrative in more detail, resorting more or less to pantomime, appropriate eye gaze is especially important. A hunter describing the shooting of a deer is likely to let his or her gaze aim down the barrel of the imaginary gun, and a golfer describing a hook shot into the woods may follow the trajectory of the ball for quite some time. One of the exercises for this chapter invites a search through a wallet for a driver's license. Such a search is likely to be accompanied by the imaginary inspection of the contents of the wallet as they are being removed.

The next chapter discusses role taking and the special application it has for depicting direct discourse. In this case, too, the eye gaze is appropriate for the imagined circumstances. The eye gaze of a doctor giving advice to the patient is likely to be downward, so as to emphasize authority, and it will be a sustained gaze, designed to instill compliance in the receiver. On the other hand, the patient, when speaking, will look up to the doctor respectfully. These attitudes, both mental and physical, will be reflected in the gaze behavior of the signer as he or she takes the role, first of the doctor, and then of the patient, so as to communicate the content of their conversation.

Chapter 9 discusses various ways in which emphasis can be added to a statement. Eye gaze can clearly play an important role here. Baker (1976a) mentions that a tall tree can be indicated by directing the gaze upward toward its branches.

If eye contact with the receiver is lacking, establishing eye contact at the exact time a sign is executed has the effect of emphasizing the sign. It is likely that other events will also be taking place, such as a frown, or a forward lean, or pursed lips, or some combination of these

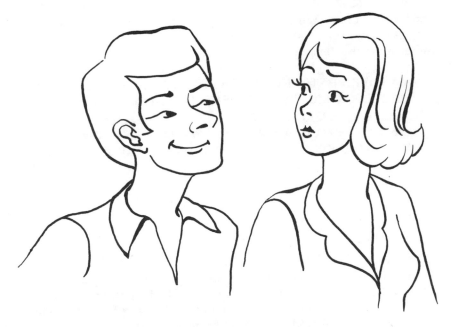

Figure 17.   Not all eye gazes are linguistic; a leer is a leer in any language.

events. Even closing the eyes, and thus effectively shutting off eye contact, can have specific semantic import in ASL. Closed eyes along with a sign like TRULY or GOOD is another way of adding emphasis. Closed eyes while telling a portion of a narrative heightens the intensity of feeling and also serves to emphasize or highlight the events being narrated.

Not all eye gazes are linguistic. A leer is a leer in any language, as Figure 17 suggests. But one must pay relatively closer attention in ASL to what one is doing with one's eyes than is the case in spoken communication. Control over eye gaze is important for communicative competence in Sign. The student of ASL should make a special effort to observe ASL users and note what they are doing with their eyes at the same time that they are communicating with their faces, hands, and bodies.

EXERCISES

Purpose

To demonstrate for students the use of eye gaze as a feature of ASL.

Instructions

The instructor may sign the following glossed sentences with indicated eye gaze and have students: 1) imitate the execution, and 2) comment on the implied meaning.

1. MAN ARRIVE STREET. TRAFFIC HEAVY. LOOK-RIGHT: LOOK-LEFT: LOOK-RIGHT; LOOK-LEFT. LOOK-LEFT (follow with eye gaze); CAR APPROACH, ZOOM PAST; LOOK-LEFT (follow with eye gaze); CAR APPROACH, ZOOM PAST. LOOK-LEFT, VACANT; LOOK-RIGHT, VACANT; DASH-ACROSS-STREET.

2. BOY WALK ON STREET, SEE QUARTER; QUICK STEP-ON. HIDE UNDER SHOE. (With head and body motionless) LOOK AROUND. (Fixating on three or four different locations). NO ONE LOOK (pointed toward signer). LOOK-DOWN (follow with eye gaze. MOVE FOOT; PICK-UP COIN.

3. I CAN'T FIND DRIVER LICENSE. TAKE OUT BILLFOLD, LOOK THROUGH (go through the motions of opening the pockets, looking into each one; pantomime removing a deck of credit cards and leaf through them, looking at each one). PUT AWAY (pantomime returning the billfold to a pocket or purse). CAN'T FIND.

4. THIS MORNING WAKE UP, WINDOW LOOK-OUT (momentarily break the eye gaze and then resume the look out the window more intently). LOOK; RABBIT IN MY GRASS; EAT HIS BREAKFAST.

5. (With eye gaze far off in the distance) MANY YEARS AGO ME WANT TRAVEL, SEE WORLD. (With direct eye contact with receiver) NOW ME WANT FIND PLACE STAY, MAKE FRIENDS, HAVE HOME.

CHAPTER 19

ROLE TAKING

One of the very effective strategies in ASL for coding a nominal or pronominal subject reference is for the signer to take the role of the person who is being referenced. The signer, with his or her own body, represents the other person. Then the signer can indicate by signs and actions exactly what it is that the other person is supposed to have done or said. Consider, for example, the following statement in English (from Hoemann, 1976), which is likely to be phrased in indirect discourse: "The doctor said that I should stay home. She said I could come to her office, but she told me not to go out for any other reason." In ASL, the signer may represent the doctor with his or her own body, taking the doctor's role, and to sign in direct discourse what the doctor said: STAY HOME. COME SEE ME, OK; OTHER OUT NO.

The economy of effort is obvious. The associated English grammatical constructions for indirect discourse are rather cumbersome. In ASL, once the signer has become the doctor, the signer can say what the doctor had to say without any further transformations.

The cues that the signer has switched roles come from the signer's body orientation, body posture, facial expression, and manner of speaking. A doctor is a person of authority. To represent the doctor as agent, the signer draws him- or herself up to a taller height, looks down at the more subordinate patient, and executes the signs with a stern, authoritative expression.

If the ASL statement had been phrased in indirect discourse (DOCTOR SAY I MUST STAY HOME), the facial expression and body stance for MUST STAY HOME would fit the speaker's mood rather than the doctor's authority.

The teacher of ASL can dramatize this device by presenting the following conversation between a child pupil and an adult teacher.

> Teacher: Where is your paper?
> Child: I don't know.
> Teacher: Stupid.
> Child: I'm sorry.

Remember that the main cues as to who is speaking are the body

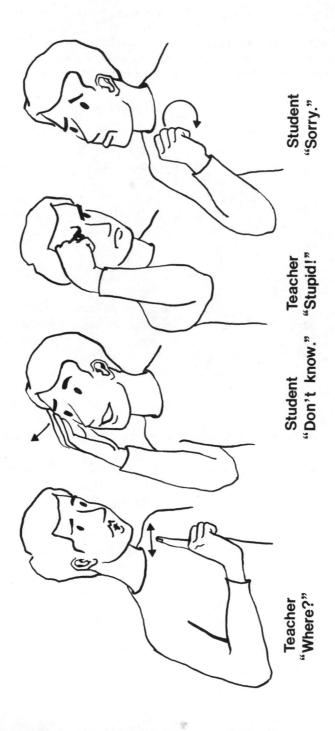

Figure 18.   Facial expression, body orientation, and eye gaze indicate whether it is the teacher or the student who is speaking.

orientation and directions of gaze, although the facial expression and body stance also are compatible with the roles. Figure 18 illustrates the compatibility of cues stemming from the facial expression, body orientation, and eye gaze. For the sake of the example, we may arbitrarily put the teacher on the left and the child on the right. When the child speaks, he faces left and looks up with a pleading expression on his face. When the teacher speaks, he faces right, looks down, and speaks with a stern facial expression.

The rapid change from one speaker to the other in the preceding example indicates that this strategy can do many more things than indicate who is speaking to whom. If a narrative involves a group of people doing things with or to each other, the signer can assume the role of each agent in turn as he or she becomes the agent of sentences in the narrative. In fact, the number of roles that can be taken in a given narrative is limited only by the narrator's ingenuity and the audience's memory.

One caution needs to be inserted for the unsuspecting student. These role changes sometimes take place very abruptly and without advance warning. The cues that signal which role is being played at the moment are sometimes subtle, too subtle, perhaps, for the uninitiated, who lack a lifetime of experience in role taking and role interpreting.

A talented deaf narrator once told the following version of "Cinderella." Cinderella brought an empty beer can to the fairy godmother. The fairy godmother touched the beer can with her magic wand, and it became a four-on-the-floor sports car. Cinderella then peeled off for the ball. The role taking that took place went as follows: 1) Cinderella brings the beer can.   2) The fairy godmother touches it with her wand.   3) The narrator registers surprise, role playing the unseen audience to the event.   4) Cinderella manipulates the stick shift and shoves it into gear.   5) The narrator signs FOUR to be sure that the real audience catches on that the carriage is really a sports car.   6) The narrator slices his right upturned hand off the left and into the distance, representing the sports car careening off to the ballroom. The entire sequence took no more than ten seconds.

To help students appreciate the efficiency and clarity of role taking as a means of communicating, the following exercise is recommended.

EXERCISE

Purpose

To give students practice in role taking as a means of indicating the agent of a statement or action.

Instructions

After the instructor has supplied the necessary vocabulary, students are to translate the following statements into ASL, using role taking and spatial organization as strategies.

1. The boy looked at his father and said, "Where are you going?"
2. The policeman said, "Get out of the car."
3. A bird flew down to eat some grain. A cat saw it. The cat watched the bird intently, crept up quietly, and pounced. The bird escaped. The cat was disappointed.
4. I went to the store and complained that my TV didn't work. The man was cross and accused me of breaking it. I said I didn't, that it wasn't my fault. But I don't think he believed me.
5. Three men went into a bar to buy a drink. The first two ordered a beer, and the third ordered a glass of milk. The first man looked at the second, and the second man looked at the first. Then both men looked at the third man and said, "Milk?" He said, "Sure, why not?"

CHAPTER 20

BREATHING AND SIGNING

Speech requires breath, and the limitation of human lung capacity and muscle control play a role in speech production. Sign has no such limitation; yet, the breathing of the signer is an aspect of the signer's physical presence that influences the way in which the signed message will be understood. Consequently, it may become a part of the nonmanual aspect of sign language productions.

For example, a narrative that gradually builds to a climax may be punctuated by a sigh of relief, followed by the denouement. The sequence might run as follows: MY BOY LOST. LOOK, LOOK, LOOK, CAN'T FIND, CAN'T FIND; FINALLY (breathe sigh of relief) FIND BOY STORE BASEMENT, PLAY WITH TOY. This might be translated into English as follows: "My boy got lost, and I looked for him everywhere but I couldn't find him; finally, to my great relief, I found him in the basement of the store playing with the toys."

A narrative involving the need to make an important decision or to take courageous action may include a deep breath just before the decisive moment or statement. As an example, a narrator might say: HARD DECIDE, HARD DECIDE (pause and relax, taking a deep breath) KNOW; MUST ACCEPT, MUST. This might be translated into English as: "The decision was really a hard one to make, but after thinking about it, I knew I had no choice but to accept."

Incidentally, the two English translations above illustrate some of the special difficulty that a translator has working from a sign language into a spoken language. How does one deal with the wealth of information that the signer is presenting by means of nonlinguistic as well as linguistic cues about his or her state of mind? The breathing behaviors of the two examples above were subjected to translation for the sake of clarifying the examples in the text. But translators who choose to do this systematically are likely to find themselves making many uncomfortable judgments about the speaker's intent.

Any ASL message that follows narrative order or includes some pantomime is likely to involve a model of the breathing behavior that is appropriate for the action. Consider, for example, a man who wishes to explain how much effort it took to push his car out of a snowdrift. As he dramatizes the physical force required, pushing against the imaginary automobile lodged in the snow, it is highly improbable that his breathing will continue without any effect from the feigned exertion. As a matter of fact, the signer is likely to puff out his cheeks and hold his breath in order to display facial and bodily cues breathing that is suitable or appropriate for the narrative.

Audible breathing, such as drawing in the breath through teeth or lips, is discussed in Chapter 9 as a stress marker. One may also breathe out through relaxed lips, even making a flubbery sound, to indicate relief, exasperation, or disgust. An approximation of a whistle is also found among deaf users of ASL for the same range of nuances as are associated with a whistle in our culture generally—something very expensive, a narrow escape, or a beautiful woman.

How important is breath control for a sign language? Not as important as eye control, and not as important in a sign language as in a spoken language. But the complex manner in which linguistic and non-linguistic features of ASL are related to one another as co-occurring events has only recently begun to be appreciated. It would be surprising if the breathing behavior of native signers while signing did not differ significantly from the breathing behavior of non-native signers. Students and teachers of ASL have the opportunity to include breathing in, breathing out, and holding the breath as a part of what they will pay attention to as they observe ASL in use.

EXERCISES

Purpose

To sensitize students of ASL to the role of breathing as a nonmanual feature of ASL.

Instructions

Students may be asked to demonstrate breathing behavior, including audible sounds, that would be appropriate for the following:

1. Mother chiding child: (Deep breath) ME ANGRY; FINISH.
2. Disgust: MAN PAINT MY HOUSE (flubber) TERRIBLE.
3. Surprise: ME WANT BUY NEW CAR (whistle) EXPENSIVE.
4. Relief: RAIN. THINK FORGET, LEAVE WINDOW OPEN. (Sigh of relief) FIND LATER, OK.
5. Determination: TOOTH HURT. MUST SEE DENTIST. DON'T WANT. (Deep breath) MAKE APPOINTMENT.

CHAPTER 21

SONG AND POETRY IN SIGN

Spending class time signing songs and poetry is desirable for a number of reasons. It involves the students in active participation, it creates some challenging problems for translation, and it invites students to consider not only the preservation of meaning in translation but also the creation of similar emotional or aesthetic effects in an audience.

The constraint that meter and end rhyme sometimes impose on translators is an especially demanding one. Some literary forms, such as the 5-7-5 syllable count of the Haiku, are all but untranslatable in Sign. In cases like this one must find in Sign a means of conveying the same impression of a willingness to conform to strict structural limitations in order to signal a specific literary function or subject matter.

Klima and Bellugi (1975b, 1976) have analyzed ASL translations of poetry and identified structural differences between poetry and prose. As an example of "internal structure" they cite a tendency to choose signs with similar handshapes. Examples of external structure include: 1) the maintaining of balance by using both right and left hands, sometimes alternately, and by overlapping the execution of signs; and 2) the creating of a "flow of movement" or a "continuity between signs." Klima and Bellugi describe another type of external structure, "external kinetic superstructure," characterized by the use of large, open, nonintersecting movements.

Churches for deaf people have garnered a great deal of experience in signing poetry and song. The Bible contains a wide variety of literary genre, and poetry is found from Genesis to Revelation. Hymnody and religious songs are an important feature of many Jewish and Christian traditions, and a robed Sign Language choir, such as is suggested in Figure 19, has graced the worship services of many congregations. Some churches have published glosses of hymns and psalms as aids for signing them in worship services (DeLaney and Bailey, 1959; Riekehof, 1976). The National Grange has recently published a song book (*Lift Up Your Hands*) of spiritual and patriotic songs (Gadling, Pokorny, and Riekehof, 1976). Religious workers with the deaf tend to appreciate the importance of ASL as their primary means of communicating with their parishoners (Pokorny, 1974).

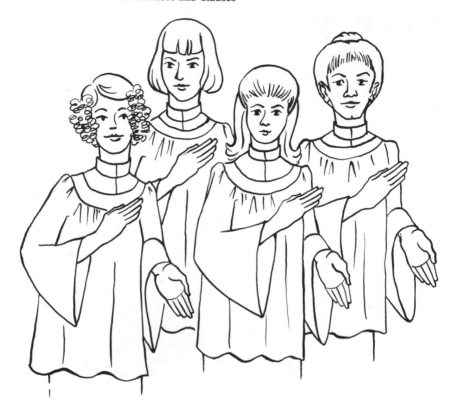

Figure 19.   A robed choir may add a great deal to the beauty of a worship service in Sign.

A high standard of professional competence and literary excellence has been set by the National Theater of the Deaf, the Detroit Sign Company, the Fairmount Theater of the Deaf (Cleveland Heights, Ohio), and the Joyce Motion Picture Company (Northridge, Cal.) in translating poetry and prose into Sign. The Gallaudet Modern Dance Group includes interpretive use of Sign as part of its performances. Modern dance is an art form that lends itself well to the incorporation of features from a sign language. Even when specific features of ASL are not discernible, the power of modern dance to communicate feeling and beauty is one of its important attractions (Figure 20). Outstanding in their field for both song and Sign is the Rock Gospel group. Films and videotapes of ASL translations of English poetry are beginning to become available from educational and commercial sources, such as the E. M. Gallaudet Memorial Library at Gallaudet College and the Joyce Motion Picture Company.

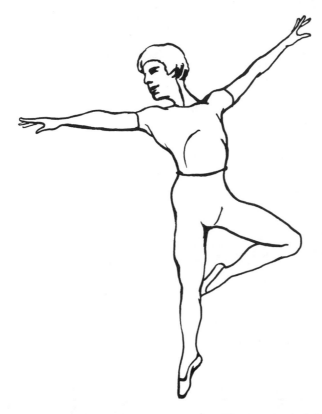

Figure 20.   Modern dance lends itself well to modifications that include features of ASL.

Most encouraging of all is the beginning of the emergence of a sign language literature. Already, a playwright, Gil Eastman (1974), and a poet, Dorothy Miles (Ruth Brown, 1977; Miles, 1977), have published literature originally conceived in Sign. Currently, the paucity of sign language literature on film and videotape is a serious handicap to the teaching of Sign, since students are completely dependent on their teacher for models of acceptable usage. Most other languages taught on college campuses have centuries of history to determine which examples of its prose and poetry are outstanding.

If all teachers of Sign would publicly call for original ASL literature, publishers would be encouraged somehow to print it, and deaf persons would be more likely to create it.

EXERCISES

(1) Purpose

To encourage students to undertake the translation of English poetry and song into Sign.

Instructions

Let each student choose a modern song from rock, country, or folk music and prepare a sign translation in class with recorded accompanyment.

(2) Purpose

To invite students to rise to the challenge confronting serious translators of poetry.

Instructions

Each of the following classes of literary material presents a special challenge to a translator. Discuss alternative solutions and adopt criteria for an acceptable translation.

1. Mother Goose—Especially useful are poems like Hickory Dickory Dock, As I Was Going to St. Ives, Jack Be Nimble, The House That Jack Built. and Row, Row, Row Your Boat.

2. Nonsense Poetry—Examples are the Jabberwocky, Mairsey Doats, and the Alphabet Song. The National Theater of the Deaf has included a Sign translation of the Jabberwocky in its repertory, and the Joyce Motion Picture Company has included Louis J. Fant's version in its offerings for sale or rent.

3. The Psalter—Students may take their favorite Psalm and attempt a Sign translation. Needless to say, if a Sign translation of the Psalter is judged to be adequate, it would be difficult to defend the thesis that ASL is a "concrete" language incapable of dealing with "abstract" concepts.

(3) Purpose

To encourage students to consider the message content of body postures and movements and to give them practice in expressing meaning nonverbally through movement and dance.

Instructions

Write down on index cards the following items and have students take turns demonstrating them with: 1) a sustained pose, or 2) a brief dance movement. Have the other members of the class write down what they think is being expressed nonverbally. If the students are equally familiar with the items to be demonstrated, the consensus among them can serve as a measure of the success of the demonstration.

1. Happiness
2. Sorrow
3. Bewilderment
4. Determination
5. Fear
6. Fatigue
7. Worry
8. Anger
9. Suspicion
10. Repose

REFERENCES

Anthony, D. A. 1971. Seeing Essential English. Vols. 1 and 2. Educational Services Division, Anaheim Union High School District, Anaheim, Cal.

Babbini, B. E. 1974. Manual Communication: Fingerspelling and the Language of Signs. University of Illinois Press, Urbana.

Baker, C. 1976a. Eye-Openers in ASL. California Linguistic Association, San Diego.

Baker, C. 1976b. What's not on the other hand in American Sign Language? Paper presented at the 12th Regional Meeting, the Chicago Linguistic Society, Chicago.

Baker, C. 1977. Regulators and turn-taking in American Sign Language discourse. In L. A. Friedman (ed.), On the Other Hand: New Perspectives on American Sign Language. Academic Press, New York.

Baker, C., and C. Padden. 1976. Studying American Sign Language as a multi-channel communication system. Paper presented at the Conference on Sign Language and Neurolinguistics, Rochester, N.Y.

Baker, C., and C. Padden. Focusing on the non-manual components of ASL discourse. Siple (ed.), Understanding Language through Sign Language Research. Academic Press, New York. In press.

Barakat, R. A. 1969. Gesture Systems. Keystone Folklore Q. 105-121.

Barakat, R. A. 1975. The Cistercian Sign Language: A Study in Non-verbal Communication. Cistercian Publications, Kalamazoo, Mich.

Battison, R. 1973. Phonology in American Sign Language: 3-D and digitivision. Paper presented at the California Linguistics Association Conference, Stanford.

Battison, R. 1974. Phonological deletion in American Sign Language. Sign Lang. Stud. 5:1-19.

Battison, R. 1976. Fingerspelled loan words in American Sign Language: Evidence for restructuring. Paper presented at the Conference on Sign Language and Neurolinguistics, Rochester, N.Y.

Battison, R. 1977. Lexical borrowing in American Sign Language: Phonological and morphological restructuring. Unpublished doctoral dissertation, University of California, San Diego.

Battison, R., and I. K. Jordan. 1976. Communication with foreign signers: Fact and fancy. Sign Lang. Stud. 10:53-68.

Battison, R., H. Markowicz, and J. C. Woodward. 1975. A good rule of thumb: Variable phonology in American Sign Language. In R. Shuy and R. Fasold (eds.), Analyzing Variation in Language. Georgetown University Press, Washington, D.C.

Bearden, C. E., and J. F. Potter. 1973. A Manual of Religious Signs. Home Mission Board of the Southern Baptist Convention, Atlanta, Ga.

Bellugi, U. 1976. Attitudes toward sign language. In A. B. Crammatte and F. B. Crammatte (eds.), Proceedings of the Seventh World Congress of the Deaf. National Association of the Deaf, Silver Spring, Md.

Bellugi, U. 1977. The signs of language. Paper presented at the National Symposium on Sign Language Research and Teaching, Chicago.

Bellugi, U., and S. Fischer. 1972. A comparison of sign language and spoken language: Rate and grammatical mechanisms. Cognition 1: 173-200.

Bellugi, U., and E. S. Klima. 1975. Aspects of sign language and its structure. In J. F. Kavanagh and J. E. Cutting (eds.), The Role of Speech in Language. MIT Press, Cambridge, Mass.

Bellugi, U., and E. S. Klima. 1976. Two faces of sign: Iconic and abstract. In S. Harnad (ed.), Origins and Evolution of Language and Speech. New York Academy of Sciences, New York.

Bellugi, U., E. S. Klima, and P. Siple. 1975. Remembering in signs. Cognition 3: 93-125.

Bode, L. 1974. Communication of agent, object and indirect object in signed and spoken languages. Percep. Mot. Skills 39: 1151-1158.

Bonvillian, J. D., and V. R. Charrow. 1972. Psycholinguistic implications of deafness: A review. Technical Report 188, Institute for Mathematical Studies in the Social Sciences, Stanford University, Stanford, Cal.

Bonvillian, J. D., V. R. Charrow, and K. E. Nelson. 1973. Psycholinguistic and educational implications of deafness. Human Dev. 16: 321-345.

Bornstein, H. 1973. A description of some current sign systems designed to represent English. Am. Ann. Deaf 118: 454-463.

Bornstein, H. 1974. Signed English: A manual approach to English language development. J. Speech Hear. Disord. 39: 330-343.

Bornstein, H., L. B. Hamilton, K. L. Saulnier, and H. L. Roy. 1975. The Signed English Dictionary for Preschool and Elementary Levels. Gallaudet College Press, Washington, D.C.

Bornstein, H., K. L. Saulnier, and L. B. Hamilton. 1976. A Guide to the Selection and Use of the Teaching Aids of the Signed English System. Gallaudet College Press, Washington, D.C.

Bragg, B. 1973. Ameslish: Our national heritage. Am. Ann. Deaf 118: 672-674.

Brown, Roger. 1977. Why are signed languages easier to learn than spoken languages? Paper presented at the National Symposium on Sign Language Research and Teaching, Chicago.

Brown, Ruth. 1977. Dorothy Squire Miles: Bard of the Deaf Theater. Deaf Am. 29: 17-18, 44.

Caccamise, F., and R. Blasdell. 1977. Reception of sentences under oral-manual interpreted simultaneous test conditions. Am. Ann. Deaf 122: 414-421.

Caccamise, F., R. Blasdell, and C. Bradley. 1977. The American Sign Language Lexicon and Guidelines for the Standardization and Development of Technical Signs. American Association for the Advancement of Science, Denver.

Caccamise, F., C. Bradley, R. Battison, R. Blasdell, K. Warren, and T. Hurwitz. 1977. A project for standardization and development of technical signs. Am. Ann. Deaf 122: 44-49.

Caccamise, F., and D. D. Johnson. Simultaneous and manual communication: Their role in rehabilitation with the adult deaf. J. Acad. Audiol. In press.

Charrow, V. R., and J. D. Fletcher. 1973. English as the second language of deaf students. Technical Report 208, Psychology and Education Series, Institute for Mathematical Studies in the Social Sciences, Stanford University, Stanford, Cal.

Charrow, V. R., and R. B. Wilbur. 1975. The deaf child as a linguistic minority. Theory Pract. 14: 353-359.

Cicourel, A. J., and R. J. Boese. 1972. Sign language acquisition and the teaching of deaf children. Am. Ann. Deaf 117: 27-33, 403-411.

Coats, G. D. 1948. Manual English. Am. Ann. Deaf 93: 174-177.

Cokely, D., and R. Gawlik. 1973. Options: A position paper on the relationship between Manual English and Sign. Deaf Am. 25: 7-11.

Cokely, D., and R. Gawlik. 1974. Options II: Childrenese as Pidgin. Deaf Am. 26: 5-6.

Cornett, R. O. 1967. Cued Speech. Am. Ann. Deaf 112: 3-13.

Coulter, G. R. 1977. Continuous representation. Paper presented at the National Symposium on Sign Language Research and Teaching, Chicago.

Covington, V. 1973a. Juncture in American Sign Language. Sign Lang. Stud. 2: 29-38.

Covington, V. 1973b. Features of stress in American Sign Language. Sign Lang. Stud. 2: 39-50.

Croneberg, C. G. 1965a. The linguistic community. In W. C. Stokoe, Jr., D. C. Casterline, and C. G. Croneberg (eds.), A Dictionary of American Sign Language on Linguistic Principles. Gallaudet College Press, Washington, D.C.

Croneberg, C. G. 1965b. Sign language dialects. In W. C. Stokoe, Jr., D. C. Casterline, and C. G. Croneberg (eds.), A Dictionary of American Sign Language on Linguistic Principles. Gallaudet College Press, Washington, D.C.

Cross, J. W. 1977. Sign language and second language teaching. Sign Lang. Stud. 16: 269-282.

Davis, A. 1966. The Language of Signs. The Executive Council of the Episcopal Church, New York.

DeLaney, T., and C. Bailey. 1959. Sing Unto the Lord: A Hymnal for the Deaf. The Lutheran Church—Missouri Synod, St. Louis.

de l'Épeé, C. M. 1776. Institution des Sourds et Muets, Par la Voie des Signes Methodiques. Chez Nyon L'Aine, Libraire, Paris.

De Matteo, A. 1976. Analogue grammar in the American Sign Language. In H. Thompson et al. (eds.), Proceedings of the Second Annual Meeting of the Berkeley Linguistic Society, Berkeley, Cal.

De Matteo, A. 1977. Visual imagery and visual analogues in American Sign Language. In L. A. Friedman (ed.), On the Other Hand: New Perspectives on American Sign Language. Academic Press, New York.

Eastman, G. C. 1974. Sign Me Alice. Gallaudet College Bookstore, Washington, D.C.

Edge, V., and L. Herrmann. 1977. Verbs and the determinant of subject in American Sign Language. In L. A. Friedman (ed.), On the Other Hand: New Perspectives on American Sign Language. Academic Press, New York.

Ellenberger, R., and M. Steyaert. 1976. A child's representation of action in American Sign Language. Paper presented at the Conference of Sign Language and Neurolinguistics, Rochester, N.Y.

Fant, L. J., Jr. 1964. Say It with Hands. American Annals of the Deaf, Washington, D.C.

Fant, L. J., Jr. 1972. Ameslan: An Introduction to American Sign Language. National Association of the Deaf, Silver Spring, Md.

Fant, L. J., Jr. 1977. Where do we go from here? Paper presented at the National Symposium on Sign Language Research and Teaching, Chicago.

Fischer, S. 1973. Two processes of reduplication in American Sign Language. Found. Lang. 9: 469-480.

Fischer, S. 1974. Sign language and linguistic universals. In C. Roher and N. Ruhet (eds.), Actes du Colloque Franco-Allemand de Grammaire Transformationelle, Vol. II. Max Niemeier Verlag, Tuebingen.

Fischer, S. 1975. Influences on word-order change in American Sign Language. In C. Li (ed.), Word Order and Word Order Change. University of Texas Press, Austin.

Fischer, S. 1976. Sign languages and Creoles. Paper presented at the Conference on Sign Language and Neurolinguistics, Rochester, N.Y.

Fleischer, L. R. 1977. Bring sign language out of the dark ages. Paper presented at the National Symposium on Sign Language Research and Teaching, Chicago.

Friedman, L. A. 1975. On the semantics of space, time, and person reference in American Sign Language. Language 51: 940-961.

Friedman, L. A. 1976. The manifestation of subject, object, and topic in American Sign Language. In N. L. Charles (ed), Subject and Topic. Academic Press, New York.

Friedman, L. A. 1977a. Formational properties of American Sign Language. In L. A. Friedman (ed.), On the Other Hand: New Perspectives on American Sign Language. Academic Press, New York.

Friedman, L. A. (ed.). 1977b. On the Other Hand: New Perspectives on American Sign Language. Academic Press, New York.

Frishberg, N. 1975. Arbitrariness and iconicity: Historical change in American Sign Language. Language 51: 696-719.

Frishberg, N. 1976. Some aspects of historical change in American Sign Language. Unpublished doctoral dissertation, University of California, San Diego.

Frishberg, N. 1977. A linguist looks at sign language teaching. Paper presented at the National Symposium on Sign Language Research and Teaching, Chicago.

Frishberg, N., and B. Gough. 1973. Time on our hands. Paper presented at the Third Annual California Linguistics Association Meeting, Stanford, Cal.

Furth, H. G. 1973. Deafness and Learning: A Psychosocial Approach. Wadsworth, Belmont, Cal.

Fusfeld, I. S. 1958. How the deaf communicate: Manual language. Am. Ann. Deaf 103: 255-263.

Gadling, D. C., D. H. Pokorny, and L. L. Riekehof. 1976. Lift Up Your Hands. The National Grange, Washington, D.C.

Goldin-Meadow, S. Structure in a manual communication system developed without a conventional language model: Language without a helping hand. In H. Whitaker and H. A. Whitaker (eds.), Studies in Neurolinguistics, Vol. 4. Academic Press, New York. In press.

Goldin-Meadow, S., and H. Feldman. 1975. The creation of a communication system. Sign Lang. Stud. 8: 225-234.

Goldin-Meadow, S., and H. Feldman. 1977. The development of language-like communication without a language model. Science 197: 401-403.

Grosjean, F., and H. Lane. 1976. Pauses and structure in American Sign Language. Paper presented at the Conference on Sign Language and Neurolinguistics. Rochester, N.Y.

Grosjean, F., and H. Lane. 1977. Pauses and syntax in American Sign Language. Cognition 5: 101-117.

Guillory, L. M. 1966. Expressive and Receptive Fingerspelling for Hearing Adults. Claitor's Book Store, Baton Rouge, La.

Gustason, G., D. Pfetzing, and E. Zawolkow. 1972. Signing Exact English. Modern Signs Press, Rossmoor, Cal.

Hawes, D. 1976. Perceptual features of the manual alphabet. Unpublished masters thesis, Bowling Green State University, Bowling Green, Ohio.

Hoemann, H. W. (ed.). 1967. Proceedings: Better Techniques of Communication for Severely Handicapped Deaf People Workshop. Catholic University Press, Washington, D.C.

Hoemann, H. W. (ed.). 1970. Improved Techniques of Communication: A Training Manual for Use with Severely Handicapped Deaf Clients. Psychology Department, Bowling Green State University, Bowling Green, Ohio.

Hoemann, H. W. 1972. The development of communication skills in deaf and hearing children. Child Dev. 43: 990-1003.

Hoemann, H. W. 1975. The transparency of meaning of sign language gestures. Sign Lang. Stud. 7: 151-161.

Hoemann, H. W. 1976. The American Sign Language: Lexical and Grammatical Notes with Translation Exercises. National Association of the Deaf, Silver Spring, Md.

Hoemann, H. W. 1977. Teaching American Sign Language: A rationale. Paper presented at the National Symposium on Sign Language Research and Teaching, Chicago.

Hoemann, H. W., and V. A. Florian. 1976. Order constraints in American Sign Language: The effects of structure on judgments of meaningfulness and on immediate recall of anomalous sign sequences. Sign Lang. Stud. 11: 121-132.

Hoemann, H. W., V. A. Florian, and S. A. Hoemann. 1976. A computer simulation of American Sign Language. Am. J. Comp. Ling. 13 (AJCL Microfiche 37).

Hoemann, H. W., and S. A. Hoemann. 1973. Sign Language Flash Cards. National Association of the Deaf, Silver Spring, Md.

Hoemann, H. W., and R. D. Tweney. 1973. Is the Sign Language of the Deaf an Adequate Communicative Channel? Proceedings of the 81st Convention of the American Psychological Association, Vol. 20. American Psychological Association, Washington, D.C.

Hoffmeister, R. J. 1977. The influence of pointing in American Sign Language Development. Paper presented at the National Symposium on Sign Language Research and Teaching, Chicago.

Hoffmeister, R. J., D. F. Moores, and R. L. Ellenberger. 1975. Some procedural guidelines for the study of the acquisition of sign languages. Sign Lang. Stud. 7: 121-137.

Ingram, R. M. 1977. Principles and Procedures of Teaching Sign Languages. The British Deaf Association, Carlisle.

Jordan, I. K. 1973. The referential communication of facial characteristics by deaf and normal-hearing adolescents. Unpublished doctoral dissertation. University of Tennessee, Knoxville.

Jordan, I. K., and R. Battison. 1976. Comparing the intelligibility of shared and foreign sign languages. In C. M. Williams (ed.), Proceedings of the Second Gallaudet Symposium on Research in Deafness: Language and Communication Research Problems. Gallaudet College Press.

Kannapell, B. M. 1974. Bilingualism: A new direction in the education of the deaf. Deaf Am. 26: 9-15.

Kannapell, B. M. 1977. The deaf person as a teacher of American Sign Language: Unifying and separatist functions of American Sign Language. Paper presented at the National Symposium on Sign Language Research and Teaching, Chicago.

Kannapell, B. M., L. B. Hamilton, and H. Bornstein. 1969. Signs for Instructional Purposes. Gallaudet College Press, Washington, D.C.

Kegl, J. A., and R. B. Wilbur. 1976. When does structure stop and style begin? Syntax, morphology, and phonology vs. stylistic variation in American Sign Language. Unpublished Manuscript.

Klima, E. S. 1975. Sound and its absence in the linguistic symbol. In J. F. Kavanagh and J. E. Cutting (eds.), The Role of Speech in Language. MIT Press, Cambridge, Mass.

Klima, E. S. and U. Bellugi. 1972. The signs of language in child and chimpanzee. In T. Alloway, L. Krames, and P. Pliner (eds.), Communication and Affect: A Comparative Approach. Academic Press, New York.

Klima, E. S., and U. Bellugi. 1974. Language in another mode. In E. Lenneberg (ed.), Language and the Brain, Developmental Aspects. Neuroscience Research Program Bulletin 12: 539-550.

Klima, E. S., and U. Bellugi. 1975a. Perception and production in a visually based language. In D. Aaronson and R. W. Rieber (eds.), Developmental Psycholinguistics and Communication Disorders. New York Academy of Sciences, New York.

Klima, E. S., and U. Bellugi. 1975b. Wit and poetry in American Sign Language. Sign Lang. Stud. 8: 203-224.

Klima, E. S., and U. Belugi. 1976. Poetry and song in a language without sound. Cognition 4: 45-97.

Klima, E. S., and U. Bellugi. The Signs of Language. Harvard University Press, Cambridge, Mass. In press.

Kuschel, R. 1973. The silent inventor: The creation of a sign language by the only deaf mute on a Polynesian island. Sign Lang. Stud. 3: 1-28.

Lane, H. 1976. The Wild Boy of Aveyron. Harvard University Press, Cambridge, Mass.

Lane, H. 1977. Notes for a psycho history of American Sign Language. Deaf Am. 30: 3-7.

Lane, H., P. Boyes-Braem, and U. Bellugi. 1976. Preliminaries to a distinctive feature analysis of American Sign Language. Cog. Psychol. 8:263-289.

Lentz, E. M. 1977. Informing the deaf about the A.S.L. structure. Paper presented at the National Symposium on Sign Language Research and Teaching, Chicago.

Liddell, S. K. 1976. An introduction to relative clauses in American Sign Language. Paper presented at the Conference on Sign Language and Neurolinguistics, Rochester, N.Y.

Liddell, S. K. 1977a. An investigation into the syntactic structure of American Sign Language. Unpublished doctoral dissertation, University of California, San Diego.

Liddell, S. K. 1977b. Non-manual signals in American Sign Language: A many layered system. Paper presented at the National Symposium on Sign Language Research and Teaching, Chicago.

Long, J. S. 1918. The Sign Language: A Manual of Signs. Athens Press, Iowa City.

Madsen, W. J. 1972. Conversational Sign Language II: An Intermediate-Advanced Manual. Gallaudet College, Washington, D.C.

Mandell, M. A. 1977a. Iconic devices in American Sign Language. In L. A. Friedman (ed.), On the Other Hand: New Perspectives on American Sign Language. Academic Press, New York.

Mandel, M. A. 1977b. Iconicity of signs and their learnability by non-signers. Paper presented at the National Symposium on Sign Language Research and Teaching, Chicago.

Markowicz, H. 1972. Some sociolinguistic considerations of American Sign Language. Sign Lang. Stud. 1: 15-41.

Markowicz, H. 1976. L'Epee's methodical signs revisited. In C. M. Williams (ed.), Proceedings of the Second Gallaudet Symposium on Research in Deafness: Language and Communication Research Problems. Gallaudet College Press, Washington, D.C.

Markowicz, H. 1977. American Sign Language: Fact and Fancy. Public Service Programs, Gallaudet College, Washington, D.C.

Markowicz, H., and J. C. Woodward, Jr. Language and the maintenance of ethnic boundaries in the deaf community. In R. Wilbur (ed.), Sign Language Research. A Special Issue of Communication and Cognition. In press.

Mayberry, R. I. 1978. Manual communication. In H. Davis and S. R. Silverman (eds.), Hearing and Deafness, 4th Ed. Holt, Rinehart and Winston, New York.

Meadow, K. P. 1972. Sociolinguistics, sign language, and the deaf subculture. In T. J. O'Rourke (ed.), Psycholinguistics and Total Communication: The State of the Art. American Annals of the Deaf, Washington, D.C.

Miles, D. 1977. Gestures. Joyce Motion Picture Co., Northridge, Cal.

Mindel, E. D., and M. Vernon. 1971. They Grow in Silence. National Association of the Deaf, Silver Spring, Md.

Moores, D. F. 1972. Communication—Some unanswered questions and some unquestioned answers. In T. J. O'Rourke (ed.), Psycholinguistics and Total Communication: The State of the Art. American Annals of the Deaf, Washington, D.C.

Moores, D. F. 1973. Gestures, signs and speech in the evaluation of programs. Sign Lang. Stud. 3: 9-28.

Moores, D. F. 1977. Issues in the utilization of manual communication. Paper presented at the National Symposium on Sign Language Research and Teaching, Chicago.

Mossel, M. N. 1956-1957. Manually Speaking. Serialized in The Silent Worker.

O'Rourke, T. J. 1972. A Basic Course in Manual Communication. Rev. Ed. National Association of the Deaf, Silver Spring, Md.

O'Rourke, T. J. 1977. The way we are. Paper presented at the National Symposium on Sign Language Research and Teaching, Chicago.

Padden, C. 1976. The eyes have it: Linguistic function of the eye in American Sign Language. In C. M. Williams (ed.), Proceedings of the Second Gallaudet Symposium on Research in Deafness: Language and Communication Research Problems. Gallaudet College Press, Washington, D.C.

Padden, C. 1977. Some contributions of research in American Sign Language toward a linguistic awareness of A.S.L. Paper presented at the National Symposium on Sign Language Research and Teaching, Chicago.

Padden, C., and H. Markowicz, 1976. Cultural conflicts between hearing and deaf communities. In F. B. Crammatte and A. B. Crammatte (eds.), Proceedings of the Seventh World Congress of the World Federation of the Deaf. National Association of the Deaf, Silver Spring, Md.

Paget, R. and P. Gorman. 1968. A Systematic Sign Language. National Institute for the Deaf, London.

Pedersen, C. C. 1977. Verb modulations in American Sign Language. Paper presented at the National Symposium on Sign Language Research and Teaching, Chicago.

Peled, T. (n.d.). A system of notation for the gesture language of the deaf. Unpublished paper, Hebrew University of Jerusalem and the Israel Institute of Applied Social Research. (Available through the Gallaudet College Library.)

Pokorny, D. 1974. The importance of sign language in worship of the deaf. In D. Pokorny (ed.), My Eyes Are My Ears. MSS Information Corporation, New York.

Riekehof, L. L. 1963. Talk to the Deaf. Gospel Publishing House, Springfield, Mo.

Riekehof, L. L. 1976. Hymns in sign language. In D. Pokorny (ed.), The Word in Signs and Wonders. Arno Press, New York.

Schlesinger, H. S., and K. P. Meadow. 1972. Sound and Sign: Childhood Deafness and Mental Health. University of California Press, Berkeley.

Siple, P. (ed.). 1978. Understanding Language Through Sign Language Research. Academic Press, New York. (Contains selected papers from the Conference on Sign Lanugage and Neurolinguistics, Rochester, N.Y., 1976.)

Siple, P. Constraints for Sign Language from Visual Perception Data. Sign Lang. Stud. In press.

Siple, P., S. D. Fischer, and U. Bellugi. 1977. Memory for non-semantic attributes of American Sign Language signs and English words. J. Verb. Learn. Verb. Behav. 16: 561-574.

Stokoe, W. C., Jr. 1960. Sign language structure: An outline of the visual communication systems of the American deaf. Studies in Linguistics, Occasional Papers: 8, University of Buffalo Press, Buffalo.

Stokoe, W. C., Jr. 1971. The Study of Sign Language. Rev. Ed. Linguistics Research Laboratory, Gallaudet College, Washington, D.C.

Stokoe, W. C., Jr. 1972. Semiotics and Human Sign Languages. Mouton, The Hague.

Stokoe, W. C., Jr. 1974. Classification and description of sign languages. In T. A. Sebeok (ed.), Current Trends in Linguistics. Mouton, The Hague.

Stokoe, W. C., Jr. 1975. The shape of a soundless language. In J. F. Kavanagh and J. C. Cutting (eds.), The Role of Speech in Language. MIT Press, Cambridge, Mass.

Stokoe, W. C., Jr., D. C. Casterline, and C. G. Croneberg. 1965. A Dictionary of American Sign Language on Linguistic Principles. Gallaudet College Press, Washington, D.C.

Supalla, T., and E. Newport. 1976. Systems for modulating nouns and verbs in American Sign Language. Paper presented at the Conference on Sign Language and Neurolinguistics, Rochester, N.Y.

Supalla, T., and E. Newport. 1978. How many seats in a chair? The derivation of nouns and verbs in American Sign Language. In P. Siple (ed.), Understanding Language Through Sign Language Research. Academic Press, New York.

Sutton, V. 1977. Sutton Movement Shorthand: Writing Tool for Research. The Movement Shorthand Society, Irvine, Cal.

Tervoort, B. T. 1968. You Me Downtown Movie Fun. Lingua 21: 455-465.

Tweney, R. D. Sign language and psycholinguistic process: Facts, hypotheses, and implications for interpretation. In D. Gerver and H. W. Sinaiko (eds.), Language, Interpretation, and Communication. Plenum Press, New York. In press.

Tweney, R. D., and H. W. Hoemann. 1973. Back translation: A method for the analysis of manual languages. Sign Lang. Stud. 2:51-72, 77-80.

Tweney, R. D. and H. W. Hoemann. 1976. Translation and sign languages. In R. W. Brislin (ed.), Translation: Applications and Research. Gardner Press, New York.

Watson, D. 1964. Talk With Your Hands. The George Banta Co., Menasha, Wis.

Wilbur, R. B. 1976. The linguistics of manual languages and manual systems. In L. L. Lloyd (ed.), Communication Assessment and Intervention Strategies. University Park Press, Baltimore.

Wilbur, R. B. American Sign Language and Sign Systems. University Park Press, Baltimore. In press.

Woodward, J. C., Jr. 1973. Implicational lects on the deaf diglossic continuum. Unpublished doctoral dissertation, Georgetown University, Washington, D.C.

Woodward, J. C., Jr. 1973c. Some characteristics of Pidgin Sign English. Sign Lang. Stud. 3: 39-46.

Woodward, J. C., Jr. 1974a. Implication variation in American Sign Language: Negative incorporation. Sign Lang. Stud. 5: 20-30.

Woodward, J. C., Jr. 1974b. A report on Montana Washington implicational research. Sign Lang. Stud. 4: 77-101.

Woodward, J. C., Jr. 1976a. Black Southern Signing. Lang. Soc. 5: 211-218.

Woodward, J. C., Jr. 1976b. Historical bases of American Sign Language. Paper presented at the Conference on Sign Language and Neurolinguistics, Rochester, N.Y.

Woodward, J. C., Jr. 1976c. Signs of change: Historical variation in American Sign Language. Sign Lang. Stud. 10: 81-94.

Woodward, J. C. Jr. 1976d. Signs of sexual behavior. Paper presented at the National Registry of Interpreters for the Deaf Conference. St. Petersburg, Fla.

Woodward, J. C., Jr., 1977. Sex is definitely a problem: Interpreters' knowledge of signs for sexual behavior. Sign Lang. Stud. 14: 73-88.

Woodward, J. C., Jr., and C. Erting. 1975. Synchronic variation and historical change in American Sign Language. Lang. Sci. 37: 9-12.

Woodward, J. C., Jr., C. Erting, and S. Oliver. 1976. Facing and hand(l)ing variation in American Sign Language phonology. Sign Lang. Stud. 11: 43-51.

Woodward, J. C., Jr., and H. Markowicz. Some handy new ideas on Pidgins and Creoles: Pidgin Sign Languages. In R. Day & D. Bickerton (eds.), Selected Papers from the 1975 International Conference on Pidgin and Creole Languages. University of Hawaii Press, Honolulu. In press.

Author Index

Subject Index

Adjectives, as plural indicators, 25
Agent — patient distinction, 67
Agent — patient networks, in cognitive constructions of deaf children, 69—70
Agent — patient representation, by role taking, 99
Allocher, 6
American Sign Language (Sign)
    "distinctive features," 7, 8
    in films and videotapes, 104, 105
    in the fine arts, 103—105
    grammar, 1, 58, 59
        importance of spatial organization to, 68
        see also Spatial organization
    lack of models of usage for, 105
    as a language, 1, 2
    linguistic analysis, 1, 2, 5—9
    native users, 57—58
    phonology, 2, 8
    in religion, 103
    sign order, 58
    signing styles, 63
    spatial organization, 58—59

Bilinguality, in English and ASL, 57
Body stance
    and imperatives, 80—81
    and indicatives, 79—81
    and interrogatives, 79—81
    as juncture marker, 87—89
    as nonmanual stress marker, 45
    and points of discussion, 68
    relationship to breathing, 102
    in role taking, 97, 99
    as temporal indicator, 74, 75
    use with ASL, 48—49, 51
Breathing, 101—102
    importance of, 102
    in narrative communication, 101—102
    as nonmanual stress marker, 28, 43, 101—102
    as temporal indicator, 77
    and translation difficulties, 101

Cheremes, 2
Cognitive capacity, in deaf children, 69—70
Compounds, 31—32
    and changes in execution, 31
    translation from English to ASL, 32
Concrete operatory thinking, 69
Conditional sentences, 83—84
Conjunctions, elimination of, 67
Contrastive analysis, 9

Dance, with ASL, 104
Designator (DEZ), 5
Detroit Sign Company, 104
Direct vs. indirect objects, distinction between, 66
Direction, indication of, 66
Distance, indication of, 66

Emotional display
    in children, 47—48
    by deaf people, 48—49
    use with ASL, 49, 51
Eye gaze, 91—94
    adding emphasis with, 93—94
        see also Stress, for emphasis in ASL
    and conversational control, 91
    importance of, 91, 94
    and pantomime, 92—93
    in pronominal referencing, 69, 92
    relationship to cognitive constructs, 69
    in role taking, 93, 99
    secretive, in surreptitious pronominal referencing, 92
    and sign space, 91
        see also Sign space, and visual acuity

Facial expression, 6, 49
    adding emphasis with, 43, 45
    and imperatives, 80—81

121

NOTES

NOTES

NOTES

NOTES

NOTES

NOTES

NOTES

NOTES